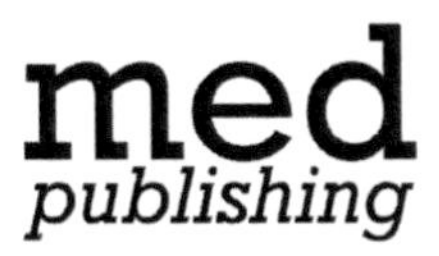

DISCLAIMER:
This publication is intended for the use of medical practitioners in the UK and not the patients. The author, editors and publisher have taken care to ensure that the information contained in this book is correct to the best of their knowledge, at the time of publication. Whilst efforts have been made to ensure the accuracy of the information presented, the author, editors and publisher cannot accept liability for information that is subsequently shown to be wrong.

ISBN 978-0-9561832-0-0

Published by Med Publishing
www.medpublishing.co.uk

Typeset by Med Publishing
Printed by Greystones Printing, Unstone Green

Contents

Foreword

On my first holiday to the Lake District I camped in Langdale and walked over to Wastdale by Sty Head Tarn. I carried an Ordinance Survey map of the Fells and a compass; but much more importantly, I also carried Alfred Wainwright's magnificent Guide to the Southern Fells. A good guide book is an enhancement to any journey. I remember the anticipation and excitement when I first opened the pages of Wainwright's Guide to the Southern Fells, which brought the Ordinance Survey map to life, even before I had set foot in the Lake District.

If the RCGP Curriculum is the equivalent my Ordinance Survey Map, then 'Becoming a GP' is the Wainwright Guide for the GP trainee.

This is not a book about short cuts to passing the MRCGP examination, rather it is a book about the journey; the journey towards becoming an excellent GP. As the learner takes their first tentative steps in General Practice, this book will guide the reader from the novice in need of further development towards excellence and mastery.

As an experienced GP and college examiner Amar Rughani demonstrates that passing the MRCGP examination is not the destination, but a consequence of being an excellent GP. His careful description of the journey calls to mind the "expert generalist" – the Master of ALL trades (and Jack of none.)

So there are no quick fixes in this book. Any fell walker will warn you to avoid taking a short cut by following the straightest line on the map. This way is sure to lead over the cliff edge. Instead, "Becoming a GP" contains a detailed description of the journey. The book sets out the way points along the road to excellence and the self assessment tools in chapter one allow the learner to find their bearings.

It is a text for the learner, but it is also a text for the trainer who guides the learner on their exciting journey. Furthermore, it can be a resource for those of us who have travelled and are still travelling the journey. Every GP will, on turning the pages of this book, find insights that resonate with their experiences and will be stimulated by the author's observations and questions. With recertification and revalidation as part of our professional lives, there is no better time for GPs to be asking ourselves where we are on our journey towards excellence.

Amar Rughani understands that the curriculum is ever changing, as patients' needs and expectations evolve and the seemingly infinite potential for health care expands, driven in large part by technological change. In this climate of rapid and sometimes revolutionary change, the book describes a structure for the learner that will form an enduring framework for a life long professional journey in which patients are presented as our teachers.

Tim Norfolk's clustering model of Relationships, Management and Diagnostics (RDMp) is a helpful framework covering the art and science of General Practice and containing at its overlapping core: professionalism. If "Relationship" is the heart of General Practice, then surely "Diagnostics" are the brain or mind and "Management", the ability to put it all together fluently in the context of primary care, is the skeleton or body. Professionalism that lies within all three areas, must be the soul of medical practice.

The insights into our behavioural traits that underpin the competences are fascinating. These traits are developed early in life and some may be behaviours that can work on to enhance and develop ourselves as the excellent GP, some positive behaviours we can work with and other behaviours we have to learn to work around.

Written in a conversational style this book is good to read, but equally good to use as a look up or for those who prefer to dip in and out. The helpful boxes of insights, questions, key notes and assessment tips should stimulate the reader and form helpful pointers to help the traveller better appreciate the landscape that is the GP curriculum.

Whilst many books are written about the MRCGP examination, most fail to inspire, focusing on "minimum competence" and promising the reader shortcuts to success. It is my hope that the reader of this book will be inspired about the lifelong journey to excellence in General Practice, in much the same way that Alfred Wainwright inspired me as a teenager planning my first trip to the Southern Fells.

Dr Mark Purvis

Director (Postgraduate GP Education) & Head of School of Primary Care
Yorkshire and the Humber Deanery

References:

The Southern Fells: Being an Illustrated Account of a Study and Exploration of the Mountains in the English Lake District: Southern Fells Bk. 4 (Pictorial Guides to the Lakeland Fells) Wainwright A.

RCGP Curriculum Statements RCGP 2007

Norfolk TD, Siriwardena AN. A unifying theory of general practice: relationship, diagnostics, management and professionalism (RDM-p) Quality in Primary Care 2009; 17, 37-47

Foreword

At the end of the 60th year of the NHS and 40 years after the inception of a professional qualification for doctors in Primary Care, we still struggle to define 'the generalist'. The recent development of a GP curriculum in 2007, defining the breadth of evidence expected of a practitioner in primary care has been a significant step forward. The curriculum is an evolving process, responding to the ever changing evidence base. There is, however, always a requirement for a practical translation of the evidence base into a 'living document' useful to the trainee, teacher and assessor alike. Ideally, this translation should also identify and explain the standard of competence that is required for GP licensing.

Amar Rughani is a practising GP, educationalist and assessor and was one of the group who developed the nMRCGP. He has adeptly provided a practical guide enabling the novice and expert alike to best implement current evidence into practice and to understand the level of performance required for the nMRCGP. 'Becoming a GP' uses examples drawn from current practice to illustrate the application of knowledge to daily clinical practice. He recognises the importance of individuals learning styles, and understands the need for trainees to develop life long learning strategies.

There is also recognition of how health teaching needs wider consideration, and encompasses the concepts of 'wellbeing' and 'health' as practical rather than abstract concepts. He positions health based teaching within a wider context where the patients' ideas of health and happiness are as important as their underlying diagnosis. The book, through a series of learning points and practical examples, illustrates the development of the trainee from a position of recognising their learning needs to achieving a competence and its application in more complex situations. This progression of learning is key to his educational philosophy.

At a time when the existence of the generalist is being challenged it is heartening that we have such an accomplished advocate. A recent quote by the political commentator, David Aaronovitch in the Times, questioned the role of holistic medicine and the generalist; "And decided that this "holistic" approach, is, in fact, code for "inexpert" *

This book reasserts the value of the GP as a generalist, and demonstrates the evidence that supports their role. It also shows a deep understanding of the core skills a GP requires to practice and the how clinical leadership is essential for the implementation of any health development. It is a welcome and influential addition to the widening literature on health care and the role of the generalist.

Dr Michael Bewick

Chair of Assessment, Royal College of General Practitioners, London

Reference:

*The Times. February 19th 2008

Preface

General practice has come a long way in the past century from being condemned as 'perfunctory work of perfunctory men' * to being the cornerstone of the NHS. The poor reputation that general practice had in its early years was to a degree, deserved. It was true that for far too long doctors could become GPs without specialist training or qualification. This prevented GPs from being respected as equals by their secondary care colleagues, who suspected (sometimes rightly) that doctors chose general practice through lack of personal capability, ambition or the availability of opportunities elsewhere.

As always, blanket statements hide important truths. For example, despite Generalism having a second-class status, many exceptional doctors learned from the experience of community practice and gave the medical profession important insights into healthcare. These included the nature and management of common diseases, the biopsychosocial dimensions of health and the art and science of the consultation.

We are now fortunate to be in a new era in which Generalism will come of age. This is 'pay back' time for general practice but not in the sense that GPs will turn the tables on their hospital colleagues. Quite the reverse because this will be an age in which the insights from system-orientated hospital practice will combine with those from person-orientated community practice to produce better doctors and better health care.

The nature of the modern world is of paradox, uncertainty, complexity and connectedness and each of these has a profound impact on medical management. Each word demands an essay in itself but suffice it to say that general practice, which is now defined through the new curriculum, prepares doctors to deal with these challenges in a way that no other specialty yet does.

General practice requires its experts to make justifiable decisions in situations of uncertainty across the whole medical spectrum and to do so repeatedly, fluently, reliably and of course, with compassion. This requires behaviour and understanding to be interconnected in ways that are explained in this book and which make General practice a discipline that is worthy of being called a specialty in its own right.

For all this talk of 'specialty', we shouldn't forget that GPs are trusted by patients because of their ability to connect with everyday life and not become distanced from it. As a profession, we have much to gain by raising the stature of general practice through raising its standards. Conversely, as professionals, we have much to lose by chasing the 'status' that specialism might bring.

The best doctors recognise the privilege of their vocation. My hope is that this book will, by guiding readers on the life-long journey of becoming a GP, help us to become the best doctors we can for our patients as well as better people along the way.

Dr Amar Rughani

Reference:

*Allbutt C. The act and the future of medicine. Times. 3rd January 1912

About the author

Amar Rughani is a full-time GP in Sheffield where he works in a large multiple-training practice, experiencing the realities of patient care and contributing to the learning of today's GP trainees.

As an educator, he is an Associate Postgraduate Dean in the Yorkshire and the Humber Deanery, where his lead roles are in the assessment of performance, appraisal and continuing professional development.

Nationally, he is a senior RCGP Examiner and was part of the group that designed and implemented the nMRCGP.

Currently, he is RCGP Blueprint clinical lead, responsible for ensuring that the separate elements of the exam work coherently. He also helped to produce the GP curriculum and is part of the RCGP group that is developing the curriculum further.

Acknowledgements

I would like to thank a number of people for the advice and support they have given me in the production of this book.

Firstly and most importantly, I wish to thank my wife Sue and my children Guy and Isabel for their advice and unfailing enthusiasm in seeing this project through. In particular I'm indebted to Guy who has been such a help that I think of him more as my co-author on this book!

For several years I have worked with my colleague and friend Tim Norfolk. His model of medical competency has helped to cluster the detail of general practice into concepts that can be more readily understood.

In assessment and education, I have had the privilege of working with a number of outstanding GPs whose ideas have shaped the curriculum and nMRCGP. These include David Sales, Neil Munro, Carol Blow, Nav Chana, Tim Swanwick and Mike Deighan. In more recent times, the development continues and I owe much to Jane Mamelok, Kamila Hawthorne, Niro Siriwardena, Charlotte Tulinius and Ben Riley for their support.

In my practice, I have learned much from the trainers and trainees and would like to thank them and in particular Ed Warren for his support of the early work on the MRCGP professional competence framework.

Abbreviations

AKT Applied Knowledge Test

BJGP British journal of General Practice

BMA British medical association

BMJ British medical journal

CbD Case-based discussion

CG Clinical governance

CKD Chronic kidney disease

COT Consultation observation tool

CPD Continuing professional development

CPR Cardio-pulmonary resuscitation

CSA Clinical Skills Assessment

EBM Evidence-based medicine

GMC General Medical Council

GMP Good Medical Practice

GPwSI GP with a special interest

IT Information technology

LMC Local medical committee

MSF Multi-source feedback

NFD Needs further development

NICE National institute of clinical excellence

OTC over-the-counter

PCO Primary care organisation

PDP Personal development plan (or learning plan)

QOF Quality outcome framework

RCGP Royal College of General Practitioners

RCT Randomised controlled trial

RDMp Relationship, Diagnostics, Management and professionalism

RNIB Royal national institute for the blind

SEA Significant event analysis

SIGN Scottish inter-collegiate guidelines network

WHO World health organisation

WPBA Workplace-based assessment

Dedication

For Dr Vijay Rughani, my dear Father and my continuing inspiration.

1 Introduction: Seeing the big picture

Why take notice of what this book has to say?

There are lots of books that offer advice on getting to the exam and you might very reasonably ask: 'Why should I take any notice of what *you* have to say?' I could sell myself by telling you that I'm an experienced examiner and have helped develop the new MRCGP. I could tell you that I contribute to the development of the curriculum. However, the most important thing about me is that I am a family doctor who is passionate about general practice and that I have spent much of my career trying to be the best doctor I can for the patients who put their trust in me. That ongoing journey has also helped me to become a better person than I once was and continues to stimulate and reward me beyond my expectations.

In this respect, I'm no different from many of my colleagues and in this book, I hope to help the next generation of GPs develop the mindset and skills that will help them and their patients to live healthy and fulfilled lives.

Preparing for the MRCGP

In this book, my aim will be to help you to be successful in the MRCGP and to assist you in the best way, which is by helping you to understand generalism well enough to perform to a high standard in the workplace. Surely, you may be thinking, an examiner will give me the inside knowledge, the shortcuts to get me through the exam so that I can get on with real life? Unfortunately there are no shortcuts and the reason is that the MRCGP does not test your ability to take tests, which in any case would be difficult to achieve because the exam uses lots of different types of test. Instead, the MRCGP tests what is really important ,i.e. your ability to do the job.

What do we mean by this? The Clinical Skills Assessment (CSA) and Applied Knowledge Test (AKT) are important and provide additional evidence of your ability in the artificial conditions of an examination. However, they are not the full story. If you think you can pass by cramming for AKT, going on a course for CSA and keeping your nose clean in training, you're pretty likely to be found out. Whether you get through or not depends not just on examiners but on the continual assessments and feedback from the people you work with.

So the bottom line is: don't look for shortcuts. This might surprise you; surely a course on the AKT and lots of practice questions would be the best way of getting through? In fact, the AKT examiners recommend that you learn through day-to-day general practice rather than 'learning to the test' and it has been shown that doctors who are doing just that (i.e. practising GPs) do better in the AKT than many trainees. Incidentally, this is a good example of why the new MRCGP is such a valid test of general practice: real GPs can pass it.

Similarly, the CSA requires no special tricks. It is a reproducible test of what happens in the consultation and the best way to prepare is to consult- - - - lots.

To pass the licensing exam you have to demonstrate to many people over a long period, that you are continually learning, improving your performance and are able to reliably achieve a specified level of performance. It's impossible to do this consistently without understanding what you're doing. Therefore, the best way to *prepare* for the MRCGP is by *performing* and this book will show you how. It is fact-light but (I hope) insight-rich and will help you to improve your understanding of general practice and more specifically, of the standard of performance that you need to achieve to comfortably get through the MRCGP.

Understanding Generalism

Generalism is complicated, difficult to define and therefore easy to underestimate. Like the piano, it is the easiest of the medical instruments to play, but the hardest to play well, so don't be fooled into thinking it is a soft option! The payback is that few specialties provide the opportunity to do so much for so many people. And yes, general practice is a *specialty* in its own right and takes an expert to do well. Let's think about the nature of this specialty in more detail.

Defining general practice has always been a struggle. This in itself must tell us something. In early days, it suggested something unflattering, for example that Generalism was a low-challenge 'dustbin' for those without talent, energy, ambition or all three. The gradual understanding of 'patient-centredness' helped us to see our discipline in terms of a focus upon the *person* rather than the disease. Later, we came to understand how Generalists need to communicate in order to achieve effective consultation outcomes.

These advances have led to GPs suggesting that what makes our specialty different from others is a focus on relationships, the communication skills of the consultation (where General practice has provided the most significant literature on the subject) and the high-quality teaching with which GP training is associated. However, we could argue that none of these features are singular to Generalism. Indeed, one of the great contributions that our specialty can make to all others, is to make these features part of the experience and values of ***all*** doctors.

If we think about what it is to be a Generalist, or indeed any specialist, it is helpful to think in terms of our *context* (where, with whom and for whom we work and the problems we are asked to deal with) and our *behaviour* (our thinking and actions in a professional situation).

It is useful to separate the two facets in order to illustrate that context will and should change, possibly more so in primary care than most other medical specialties. On the other hand, the behavioural base of our discipline is likely to remain relatively stable. This book describes the behavioural base (what we call our 'competencies') in detail. Mastering these competencies will help you to perform well for the exam but more importantly, to continue to perform throughout independent life even when the context of general practice inevitably changes.

Although the environment will change, there are some contextual features that characterise our specialty and are worth trying to understand because they are likely to remain important. I've selected three (**C**omplexity, **U**ncertainty & **P**artnership) to examine in more detail.

Complexity

Complexity implies the presence of many interconnected parts. All initiates to Generalism become used to plurality or the presence of multiple components, which at one level may simply be the wide range of medical conditions with which the GP may be faced. However, complexity is not simply plurality but is the **connection, integration and interaction** between parts. Engaging with complexity is a high-order cognitive ability, requiring considerable attentiveness, perception and understanding. The GP curriculum (the first our specialty has had) at last gives us a framework for learning about connections. Here are some examples of complexity in action:

- GPs do not simply deal with medical conditions but also engage with broader notions of health (rather than illness), with problems rather than just diseases and with management options that are of greater scope than drug treatments or complementary therapies.
- By considering health more broadly, GPs don't think of the mind and body as being separate from each

other, but use the interconnectedness of both. This helps us to value and use thoughts and perceptions as well as information on bodily function when we explore problems, make professional judgements and facilitate improvement.

- In clinical terms, complexity may mean an appreciation of the implications of co-morbidity (how coexistent symptoms, diseases and possible treatments impact upon each other) and how this might be anticipated and addressed.

- Complexity also operates when GPs recognise and make use of the social connections that influence the patient's health. These include the patient, the other people within the patient's social and cultural grouping and more widely, the influences of society, which includes the influence of health professionals.

What are the implications for the learning journey? It means that we should never regard any experience, learning, situation or problem as being entirely simple or isolated. To do so is to miss important opportunities to make connections. As *students*, we should learn that the different sections of the curriculum do not stand in isolation but are integrated and have effects on each other. As *practitioners*, we should learn how seemingly innocent physical, psychological and social cues can be the early signs of more significant problems. We should also learn how connections between seemingly unrelated pieces of information can allow us to recognise important patterns at an early stage.

Uncertainty

It is said that nothing is certain except death & taxes....and perhaps in the future even death may become optional! It is interesting that as society moves away from traditional certainties such as faith in religion or trust in professionals, it takes refuge in proxies for certainty such as rights, accountability and the exercise of control. Medicine, in part reflecting this movement, has developed an evidence-base paradigm that we could argue is an attempt to control uncertainty.

Like all frameworks, EBM cannot represent the whole truth although it does provide an explicit structure that can be used to educate, inform, direct, ration and measure the application of healthcare. However, in general practice uncertainty is inherent in the work that we do and a full hospital diagnostic workup or EBM are not routinely available to rescue (some would say distract?) us. With patients, there may be uncertainty over the diagnosis and more broadly, how best to manage the problem given the particular circumstances. These crucial judgements are only partly assisted by evidence-based medicine and a large part of GP expertise lies in the ability to use a resource bank of experiences from medical and non-medical contexts. In situations of uncertainty, perhaps where the problem is evolving or has never been encountered before, we rely upon the bells of our prior experience and knowledge of probability to ring in order for patterns to be recognised or events to be anticipated in a sophisticated way that reduces the risk that uncertainty represents.

Although it seems strange, uncertainty can improve our capacity to make optimum judgements. How? By indicating the limits of certainty, signposting uncharted territory that may prompt us to learn and by giving appropriate weight to the available options. Also, uncertainty helps to improve our thinking by encouraging us to make connections between bits of information in an effort to come up with lower-risk strategies to deal with a problem than we might otherwise have thought of. As we can see, uncertainty and complexity (making connections) are thereby related.

In our learning journey, we should value uncertainty and sensitise ourselves to it, for example by recognising the discomfort that it causes and using it to prompt questions such as 'What did I feel unsure of and does this matter?' In this way, uncertainty should be a routine and lifelong spur to learning.

Partnership

Partnership is a relationship between individuals or groups that is characterized by cooperation and mutual responsibility in an effort to achieve a specified goal. In our age, we are moving from compliance, where doctors tell and others obey, to concordance where there is a meeting of minds and a sharing of understanding and responsibility. Communication skills have helped to undo the harm caused by the disease-orientated approach to patient encounters. However, we are still at an early stage in the appreciation of the implications of partnership. Let's consider two facets of this.

Firstly, within the consultation we are becoming more adept at probing the patient's health beliefs and sharing appropriate management options. However, by definition partnership has at least two parties and relatively little is done to empower the patient toward greater self-sufficiency or to discuss what shared responsibility might mean from the patient's perspective beyond the rather trite concordance with prescribed medication.

Secondly, partnership is a mindset as well as a contract. We work in partnership with colleagues as well as with patients and the intention is to collaborate. For this to happen there must be a mindset of mutual respect and understanding of each other's abilities and capacity to contribute, as well as a commitment to provide the *opportunity* to contribute. We might argue that there is no equality of opportunity without the *differences* between us being valued and harnessed. In other words, equality and diversity must progress hand in hand. In practical terms, we should ask ourselves questions such as:

- 'How can I encourage my patient to wish to be my partner for this problem and for future problems?'
- 'Who else might have a view or might legitimately wish to be involved in managing this problem?'
- 'What can others add to this enterprise, even (perhaps *especially*) those people whose views I disagree with and how can I get them involved?'

In terms of our learning journey, we can summarise CUP as follows:

- Complexity: is an **opportunity** to make connections
- Uncertainty: is an **unsettled feeling** that we should not ignore but use as a prompt to learn and be creative with problem-solving.
- Partnership: is an **offer** that we should make far more often to the people we work for and with.

Who is this book for?

This book is intended to help the learning journey; performance assessment is a guest at the table of education and should enrich the conversation, not spoil the meal. By illustrating the GP competencies required for licensing, this book provides a common language that should help trainees and educators to have better-informed conversations that allow insight into performance to be improved. As a result, learning plans can be targeted to the most appropriate areas and pitched to the most appropriate level of difficulty. The latter is important, because many of the GP competencies cannot be achieved until late in training and it is counter-productive to suggest or assume that they can be mastered early on.

The book is also intended to help assessors, both those who have a responsibility for GP assessment and for trainees who wish to use their self-assessment skills to drive their learning. The book gives numerous examples of assessment tips but more importantly, it provides a basis for assessors in all components of the nMRCGP to develop their understanding of the licensing standard that is being assessed (see page 8).

What is learning for?

I've said that this book is intended to help us to learn, so it is worth asking what exactly learning is for. We all have our own response to this, but at one level the purpose of our learning (in our professional context) is in order to improve our professional performance.

The following equation, which is explored in greater depth in the chapter on 'Fitness to practise' (page 203), helps us to understand the factors underlying improvement in performance:

d performance = d (insight x motivation x application x opportunity)

d (delta) represents change.

Insight can be improved by the following mechanism:

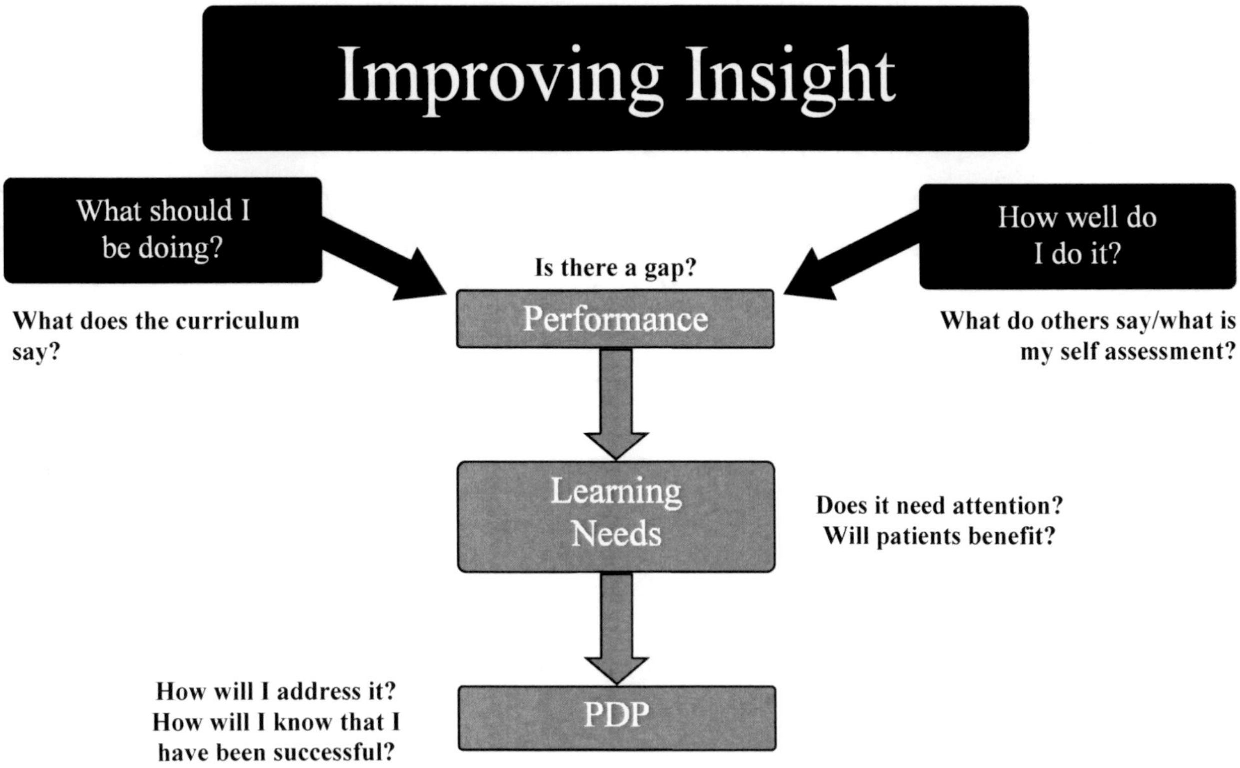

Improving Insight

What should I be doing?

What does the curriculum say?

Is there a gap?

Performance

How well do I do it?

What do others say/what is my self assessment?

Learning Needs

Does it need attention?
Will patients benefit?

How will I address it?
How will I know that I have been successful?

PDP

The crucial stage is to recognise and to interpret the gap between current performance and the level of performance that is required. This book describes the competencies and the standards so that this gap can be made more explicit and therefore discussed more productively.

Motivation is mentioned and at this stage of your career, the motivation may simply be to get through the exam. However, what about when the exam is behind you? It's worth thinking about your deeper motives and again there are no rights and wrongs. Some doctors are motivated by vocation, others by status or income and many by a combination of the three. As the equation shows, if our motivation suffers then so will our performance. Deeper motivations can't be easily changed, but if we are aware of them, we can nurture what's important and change the balance if we need to. For example, we might maintain motivation by seeking to be inspired by those whose values we admire or we might undertake work that improves our status (e.g. self-esteem) but doesn't earn income.

Looking more broadly we might say that 'performing' isn't just about being a better medic, it's about being a better person. However, is that relevant to us as GPs?

I'd say 'yes' because our expertise lies in our ability to help others make choices that are right for them in situations that are important, but uncertain. We can't do that without caring about and trying to understand people and what distresses them. To that end, we need to be better people not just better technicians. It's worth remembering that competence is not a big issue for our patients. For them, competence is a given. However, what they hope for and what they really value is our human compassion. Compassion is not a 'competency' that can be faked to get through an exam. It is a fragile virtue, but one that we know is part of the doctor's make-up when they continue to care about their patients, despite the stresses of their working environment and own lives.

'Becoming a GP', is not simply about the destination of becoming a licensed general practitioner, but about a learning journey that continues throughout life. As the philosopher Alan Watts said, life is not about some distant goal (an exam, retirement or even enlightenment) but about enjoying and making the most of each day along the path. That, he says, is why composers write symphonies, not just final movements! In a similar way, the MRCGP looks at how trainees engage with the learning journey, continually engaging with life, reflecting on their experiences and applying their insights to practice.

What do patients need?

Patients have increasing access to high quality sources of information, so doctors are less important as content experts than they used to be. Paradoxically, far from reducing the need for a doctor's advice, GPs are needed more then ever to help the patient make sense of the information and to put it in the context of their lives so that the best choices can be made. This means that patients need *guidance*, not given paternalistically but offered in a way that respects the patients desire (or lack of desire) to share in decision-making.

What do trainees need?

In order to guide patients, GPs need to be good at evaluating situations and helping others to understand and act. Although GPs also have some practical skills, our main expertise is in the development and use of our intelligence. In broad terms, let's think about two manifestations of this. *Cognitive* intelligence is mainly concerned with our ability to interpret information and to reason. Just as importantly, *emotional* intelligence concerns our 'feeling' mind especially our self-awareness and motivations, our understanding of other people's emotions and of how to manage relationships. The thrust of GP training is directed at developing both forms of intelligence.

So where do we find out what needs to be learned?

First and most importantly, the knowledge skills and attitudes that GPs require are laid out in the RCGP curriculum. The curriculum can look overwhelming, but it isn't if we remember that the basis is described in the **core curriculum statement 'Being a General Practitioner'**. The core statement has 9 principal areas as shown in the table below. The first 6 are called 'domains' and the last 3 are called 'essential features'.

In addition to the core statement there are many other curriculum statements. However they should not be thought of as being separate stand-alone areas of general practice. Their purpose is really to illustrate the ideas within the core curriculum. For example, a 'holistic approach' from the core curriculum (such as the impact of a problem on the patient's life) will manifest itself differently in a young adult with earache compared to a mother with terminal ovarian cancer. These differences are illustrated by the curriculum statements and help us to understand what the core curriculum means by 'holism'.

For the MRCGP, the domains and essential features of the core curriculum statement have been translated into 12 competency areas which we call the **competence framework**. The relationship between this framework and the curriculum is as follows:

The Curriculum:	Related MRCGP competency areas:
Primary care management	Clinical management Working with colleagues and in teams Primary care administration and IM&T
Person-centred care	Communication & consulting skills
Specific problem-solving skills	Data gathering and interpretation Making a diagnosis/making decisions
A comprehensive approach	Managing medical complexity
Community orientation	Community orientation
A holistic approach	Practising holistically
Contextual features	Community orientation
Attitudinal features	Maintaining an ethical approach to practice Fitness to practise
Scientific features	Maintaining performance, learning and teaching

Why translate the curriculum?

The core curriculum was written in order to explain the essence of being a GP. It contains many ideas, but was not designed to specify the behaviours that doctors must have in order to pass the licensing exam. This is why a translation was needed. The competence framework doesn't represent the entirety of the curriculum and to understand each of the 12 assessment areas properly, you need to read about the area of the curriculum to which it is related, as shown in the table.

By having behaviours that are specified, trainees know what they are expected to do for the MRCGP and assessors to know what to look for.

What is the structure of the competence framework?

Each of the 12 areas in the framework is further broken down into a number of themes which are separate from each other. For example,' Managing medical complexity' contains themes on:

- Managing several problems together.
- Assessing and managing clinical risk
- Health promotion

Each theme is itself developed from a lower level in the 'needs further development' column to an 'excellent' level on the right-hand side. If you look at the chapters in this book, each theme is represented by an arrow that illustrates this progression. For example:

Needs Further Development	Competent	Excellent	
Treats patients, colleagues and others equitably and with respect for their beliefs, preferences, dignity and rights.	Recognises and takes action to address prejudice, oppression and unfair discrimination within the self, other individuals and within systems.	Actively promotes equality of opportunity for patients to access health care and for individuals to achieve their potential.	2

This has been done so that trainees can see the trajectory of learning and can see how to improve their performance over time. Don't be fooled by the terminology, though. The lower-level of 'needs further development' is taxing and it is expected that most trainees will not be able to perform above this level until late on in training. It also carries with it the obligation on the trainer to offer feedback on how performance can be improved to reach the 'competent' level and beyond.

So what is good enough for licensing?

The standard required for licensing is described by the middle column labelled 'competent', which is short for 'competent for independent practice'. To achieve this licensing standard, trainees need to demonstrate the behaviours in the first column **and** the second column. The final column (excellent) is there to provide goals for those who are still in training but are already achieving the 'competent' standard in that area of performance. It also describes the trajectory of learning beyond GP training and is therefore valuable as it informs the professional development of all GPs.

Where are the 12 assessment areas tested in the MRCGP?

All 12 assessment areas are tested continually through workplace-based assessment. Most of them are also tested in the other two examination components. For example, clinical decision-making and interpersonal skills and attitudes are tested in CSA and the knowledge base of general practice and how it is applied, is tested through the AKT.

But what does it all *mean*?

Seeing the wood from the trees

Around now, you may well be feeling overwhelmed with frameworks, domains, competencies and so on, but hang on because we will now try to see the wood from the trees!

First, a word of advice: the rest of this chapter contains a lot of information and ideas which help us to understand the complexity of GP performance, and the ways in which it might be analysed for assessment and training purposes. It is not an easy read but becomes more understandable and useful as the reader becomes familiar with the book. It is therefore well worth revisiting this part of the book periodically.

As we've seen, the MRCGP is designed to test the curriculum and it does so by using the competence framework. The language of the framework is extensive but in it, there are a large number of job-related competencies and a number of deeper features which in this book I have called our 'DNA'. The term should not be taken too literally as these features are ***not immutable*** but can be developed through training and education.

The job-related competencies and the deeper features can be clustered into a 'wood' which most GPs find easy to recognise. The reason that we have all the trees (the detail of the competency framework) rather than just the wood is that the trees give us the anchor points we need in order to help us learn and in order to gauge our performance.

So how do we see the wood? The method used in this book is to bring the 12 areas of the competency framework into 4 clusters. In recent years, Tim Norfolk has developed a clustering model of medical competence called RDMp which is applied to the competence framework as shown below in Figure 1.

- **Relationship**: the doctor's ability to understand and develop human relationships principally with patients, families, colleagues and teams.
- **Diagnostics**: the doctor's ability to problem-solve particularly within a clinical context.
- **Management**: the doctor's ability to manage issues ,events, relationships and him/herself over time.
- **Professionalism**: the attitude that the doctor has about the responsibilities of the job, expressed through the level of respect and commitment demonstrated for people, professional guidelines and duties.

Figure 1: RDMp

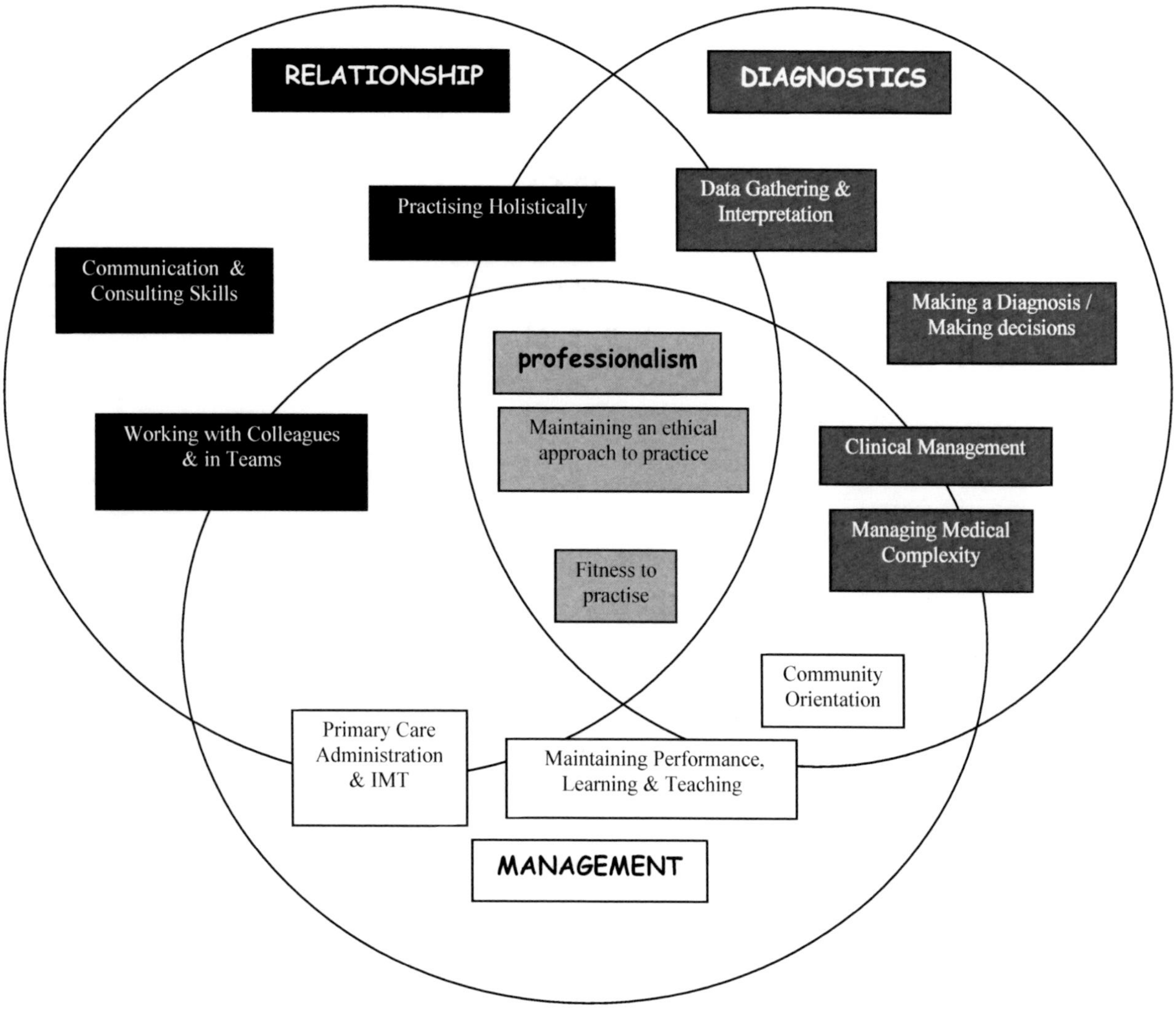

RELATIONSHIP
DIAGNOSTICS
Practising Holistically
Data Gathering & Interpretation
Communication & Consulting Skills
Making a Diagnosis / Making decisions
professionalism
Working with Colleagues & in Teams
Maintaining an ethical approach to practice
Clinical Management
Managing Medical Complexity
Fitness to practise
Community Orientation
Primary Care Administration & IMT
Maintaining Performance, Learning & Teaching
MANAGEMENT

Seeing the deeper features

Amongst the text of the word pictures of the competency framework, lie hints of deeper features. We recognise that they are present, although they are not stated explicitly. These deeper features are important because:

- They bring items of performance together in a way that we can make sense of. This is similar to the RDMp clustering idea that we have just discussed. Both methods are ways of having an overview of performance that allows important links to emerge. This then allows further training/assessments to be appropriately and efficiently targeted.
- Deeper features have prognostic importance. If they are present, then doctors are more likely to train successfully. Just as importantly, trainees can adapt to changes in their jobs over the years. If the deeper features are *not* present, it may be very difficult to do this and doctors may become poorly-performing.
- Each of the deeper features manifests itself in a large number of different contexts. Therefore, each one that is mastered can help trainees to perform well in a large number of job-related areas.

Screening for performance

We've discussed how to see the wood from the trees, but how do we bring these ideas together in a practical way? On the following pages, there are four screening forms one for each of the four RDMp clusters. In each form there is a top section from the competence framework, a middle section of deeper features and a bottom section to summarise the interpretation. **These forms can be downloaded** from www.medpublishing.co.uk

<table>
<tr><td colspan="3">Shaded areas may not be evident until the final year of training</td><td colspan="4">Please grade the trainee in comparison with doctors at the same stage of training</td><td rowspan="2">Unable to grade</td><td rowspan="2">Concerns?</td></tr>
<tr><td colspan="3"></td><td>Below expectations</td><td>Border line</td><td>Meets expectations</td><td>Above expectations</td></tr>
<tr><td rowspan="10">Relationship</td><td rowspan="5">Communication and consultation skills</td><td>Explores patient's agenda and ideas, concerns & expectations</td><td></td><td></td><td></td><td></td><td></td><td></td></tr>
<tr><td>Recognises the impact of the problem on the patient's life</td><td></td><td></td><td></td><td></td><td></td><td></td></tr>
<tr><td>Works in partnership to negotiate a plan</td><td></td><td></td><td></td><td></td><td></td><td></td></tr>
<tr><td>Explores what the patient has understood from the consultation (shaded)</td><td></td><td></td><td></td><td></td><td></td><td></td></tr>
<tr><td>Flexibly and efficiently achieves consultation tasks (shaded)</td><td></td><td></td><td></td><td></td><td></td><td></td></tr>
<tr><td rowspan="2">Practising holistically</td><td>Understands the patient's socio-economic/cultural background</td><td></td><td></td><td></td><td></td><td></td><td></td></tr>
<tr><td>Recognises the impact of the problem on family/carers</td><td></td><td></td><td></td><td></td><td></td><td></td></tr>
<tr><td rowspan="2">Working with colleagues and in teams</td><td>Works co-operatively with team members, using their skills appropriately</td><td></td><td></td><td></td><td></td><td></td><td></td></tr>
<tr><td>Communicates proactively with team members (shaded)</td><td></td><td></td><td></td><td></td><td></td><td></td></tr>
</table>

Deeper features are shown below. Ring any that apply

POSITIVE	**NEGATIVE**
• Non-judgemental, shows interest and understanding. • Encourages contribution	• Makes assumptions, authoritarian. • Lacks warmth in voice/manner
• Uses open questions, adjusts questioning • Expresses ideas clearly.	• Uses too many closed questions • Unable to adapt language.. • Unclear when communicating
• Good non-verbal behaviour	
• Delegates appropriately	• Shows favouritism
• Gives constructive feedback & support	• Critical, confrontational
• Collaborates	• Gives little support

Summary & interpretation:

Action:

Shaded areas may not be evident until the final year of training			Please grade the trainee in comparison with doctors at the **same** stage of training				Unable to grade	Concerns ?
			Below expectations	Border line	Meets expectations	Above expectations		
Diagnostics	**Data gathering and interpretation**	Takes a history, examines and investigates systematically & appropriately						
		Elicits important clinical signs & interprets information appropriately						
		Makes appropriate use of existing information about the patient's problem.						
	Making a diagnosis/ making decisions	Addresses problems that present early and in an undifferentiated way by integrating information in order to aid pattern recognition						
		Uses time as a diagnostic tool.						
		Decides what is probable and uses this to aid decision-making						
		Makes or excludes important diagnoses						
		Revises hypotheses in the light of additional information.						
		Thinks flexibly around problems, generating feasible solutions						
	Clinical management	Formulates appropriate management plans in line with best practice						
		Varies management options in response to changing circumstances.						
		Refers appropriately and co-ordinates care with other professionals						
		Provides continuity of care for the patient rather than just the problem						
	Managing medical complexity	Simultaneously manages acute and chronic problems						
		Tolerates uncertainty where appropriate						
		Communicates risk effectively to patients and involves them in its management to the appropriate degree						
		Encourages health promotion						

Deeper features are shown below. Ring any that apply

POSITIVE	NEGATIVE
• Identifies key issues • Elicits necessary detail • Aware of appropriate options	• Fails to explore important cues/overlooks important issues • Suggests too narrow a range of options
• Shows sound/systematic judgment	• Random/disorganised
• Tries to think around an issue • Open to new ideas/possibilities	• Makes immediate assumptions • Dogmatic

Summary & interpretation:

Action:

Shaded areas *may not be evident until the final year of training*			Please grade the trainee in comparison with doctors at the **same** stage of training				Unable to grade	Concerns?
			Below expectations	Border line	Meets expectations	Above expectations		
Management	**Primary care administration and IMT**	Uses the primary care organisational and IMT systems routinely and appropriately						
		Uses the computer during the consultation whilst maintaining rapport with the patient.						
		Keeps good medical records						
	Community orientation	Identifies important characteristics of the local community that might impact upon patient care						
		Encourages patients to appropriately use the community resources.						
		Uses resources cost-effectively						
	Maintaining performance, learning and teaching	Critically appraises guidelines and research evidence to inform decision-making.						
		Keeps up-to-date and shows commitment to addressing learning needs						
		Participates and learns from audit and significant event reviews						
		Completes learning cycles and routinely learns from reflection						
		Contributes to the education of students and colleagues						

Deeper features are shown below. Ring any that apply

POSITIVE	**NEGATIVE**
• Thinks ahead, plans effectively	• Fails to think ahead, plan and think about knock-on effects
• Prioritises information / time appropriately	• Unable to cope with the unexpected
• Co-ordinates activities	• Disorganised
• Able to juggle competing demands	
• Delegates effectively & demonstrates leadership when appropriate	
• Delivers on time	• Misses reasonable deadlines
• Regularly updates skills	• Doesn't have a system for keeping up to date

Summary & interpretation:

Action:

Shaded areas may not be evident until the final year of training			Please grade the trainee in comparison with doctors at the **same** stage of training				Unable to grade	Concerns?
			Below expectations	Border line	Meets expectations	Above expectations		
Professionalism	**Maintaining an ethical approach to practice**	Shows awareness of own values, attitudes and ethics and how these might influence professional behaviour.						
		Identifies and discusses ethical conflicts						
		Shows respect for others						
	Fitness to practise	Understands and maintains awareness of the GMC duties of a doctor						
		Responds to complaints appropriately						
		Is organised, efficient and takes appropriate responsibility						
		Deals appropriately with stress						
		Maintains a healthy work-life balance						

Deeper features are shown below. Ring any that apply

POSITIVE	NEGATIVE
• Demonstrates respects for others	• Lacks sufficient respect for others
• Positive/enthusiastic when dealing with problems	• Treats issues as problems rather than challenges
• Able to admit mistakes/learn from them	• Avoids taking responsibility for poor decisions/ideas
• Committed to equality of care for all	• Shows favouritism
• Backs own judgment appropriately	• Is tentative when explaining decisions/actions became tense or agitated
• Remains calm/under control	
• Uses strategies to deal with pressure/stress	
• Rarely loses sight of wider needs of situation	• Shifts focus largely to immediate worries/needs
• Recognises own limitations and can compromise	• Becomes defensive or uncompromising
• Able to seek help when necessary	• Inappropriately tries to deal with situation alone

Summary & interpretation:

Action:

Using the performance screening forms

In the **top section**, working from left to right and using the *Relationship* form as an example, we see:

1. The cluster area (relationship)
2. The relevant performance areas from the competence framework (communication & consulting skills, practising holistically, working with colleagues and in teams)
3. The key word pictures for each of the performance areas

There is a rating scale that can be used by assessors or by trainees for self-assessment. The wording of the scale suggests that comparisons are made with doctors at the same stage of training. For doctors at the *end* of training, the standard will be the 'competent for licensing' standard described in the word pictures that you will find in the large arrows of this book. For doctors at an earlier stage of training, the expected standard will be either at the level described by 'needs further development' or between and this and the 'competent' level.

Some competencies are more advanced and therefore unlikely to be developed until late on in training and these are shaded *grey* on the form.

In the **middle section**, the deeper features are listed with positive ones on the left and negative ones on the right. Positive behaviours need to be seen repeatedly and in a variety of contexts if we are to be sure that they are truly embedded and not just a fluke. The negative behaviours should not be thought of as being 'one strike and your out' offences but if any of them are seen, they should not be ignored. If a negative behaviour occurs once, it should be noted. If it is seen again, it should be regarded as a red flag and should prompt us to be concerned and to explore this area of performance in more detail.

In the **bottom section**, the summary and interpretation can be written after which any action points can be noted. The *interpretation* may include any learning needs that have been identified. The *action* might include any further training or assessment that might be required.

How are these ideas brought together in this book?

Being joined up

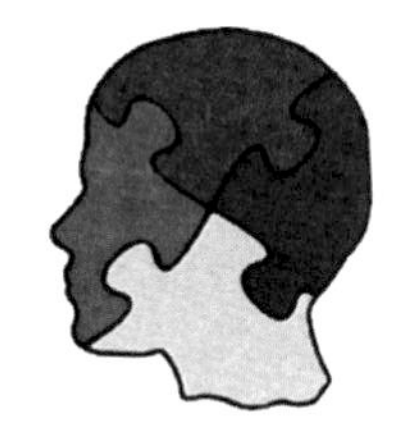

General practice can't ever be defined but by describing certain behaviours in detail, important elements can be visualised and understood.. The jigsaw picture on the right appears regularly through the book to remind learners and assessors that the detail is there to help the connections and thereby the bigger picture to be seen. This section goes on to explain these connections.

The competence framework is the backbone

As we discussed earlier, to become a GP we have to learn to use our cognitive and emotional intelligence much better than we have done before. This requires us to develop our understanding and insight. In this book, the competence framework is the backbone that is used to develop this understanding. The competencies are the building blocks of performance and lots of methods are used in the book to help readers understand not just the competencies, but the *connections* between them that help novices to become GPs.

The competence framework is presented in clusters

Each of the 12 performance areas of the framework has its own chapter. The chapters are arranged in four sections based on RDMp and at the start of each of these sections, there is a short chapter that explains why and how the performance areas in that cluster belong together.

In each performance area, there are many word pictures that describe the competencies. *It is very important that you don't look upon the competencies as being separate and unrelated items of behaviour.* If you did, you might be tempted to think that becoming a GP was simply a matter of ticking off the list of competencies.

The competencies are interconnected

The competencies are integrated at a number of levels and fit together in ways which I will illustrate using an example from the 'Communication and consultation skills' area of the framework (chapter 3 page 27).

Firstly, the competencies are arranged in **themes** in the grey arrows, with each theme being numbered. Within each theme, the competencies are placed in a sequence from left to right that illustrates the same type of behaviour but at different levels of development. For example:

'Achieves the tasks of the consultation but uses a rigid approach' is a basic level skill.

The next step up is ' flexibly and efficiently achieves consultation tasks, responding to the consultation preferences of the patient'

As you can see the second is in the same ballpark but is developed from the first and is more advanced.

Secondly, the themes are collected in 12 separate performance **areas**. Each of these has more than one theme within it, but all the themes relate to the same area of performance. In the communication and consulting skills area, there are separate themes relating to understanding the patient's thoughts, negotiating a management plan and making explanations. So, attending to the competencies helps you to master the theme which in turn helps you to master the area of performance.

Thirdly, the **areas are clustered** under the headings of RDMp.

This clustering helps us to understand how the performance areas themselves are not separate from each other but are integrated within clusters and how mastery of one member of a cluster can help us to master the whole group. Likewise, if we have problems mastering one member, we may have problems with the other members of the cluster.

To use the example of communication and consultation skills, we can see from figure 1 that this domain sits with 'practising holistically' and 'working with colleagues and in teams'. These belong to the R or 'Relationship' cluster of RDMp. Thus if we have problems with communication skills in the consultation, there is a possibility that we may also have problems with working with colleagues and team members.

Alternatively, if our problem is only with patients, we might ask what it is that stops us from being able to communicate with patients as well as we do with say a colleague (or indeed vice versa!). This is because at root we are drawing on the same range of verbal and non-verbal skills when communicating with patients, colleagues or any other member of the team.

This may sound pretty obvious but let's take other examples. 'Practising holistically' requires us to explore the impact of the patient's problem on their life. Seeing its position within Relationship helps us appreciate the fact that holism is going to be difficult to practise if we don't have the skills to develop a relationship with a patient, take an active interest in them and use communication skills to explore the impact of the problem. In the other direction, digging deeper into the patient's problem, which is what holism requires, actually helps to develop our communication skills because by behaving holistically we learn to find ways of helping patients to talk about various facets of their problem and to disclose sensitive information.

Do you notice from figure 1 that Holism overlaps with the Diagnostics field? This is because the exploration/ assessment we make of the link between the patient's problem and their life clearly requires diagnostic skill in the same way as, say, exploring the patient's past history alongside their current presentation.

Interesting, isn't it? Can you think of examples of your own?

Performance can be quickly and repeatedly screened

Using the screening forms shown earlier in this chapter, performance can be repeatedly gauged throughout training both by assessors and by learners themselves. One approach is as follows:

1. The first step is to conduct a brief screen of performance using the screening forms. The screening forms represent the four RDMp clusters and it is worth screening all four areas rather than one at a time as the clusters are interrelated and affect each other as shown in figure 1.

2. The second step is to look for links between related areas. The material that has been brought together in each form can help you with this. To take an example from the screening form for Diagnostics, if a doctor routinely over-investigated, we might mark them down on the following competency:

   'Takes a history, examines and investigates systematically & appropriately'

   We might also expect such a doctor to have difficulty with the competency:

   'Tolerates uncertainty where appropriate'

   If there was a mismatch in performance between the two, this might prompt further discussion. For example, if the doctor was over-investigating and yet was thought to be tolerating uncertainty, we might ask whether we need to look more closely at the latter.

3. The third step is to look at the deeper features. How do these correlate with what has been shown from the competency rating? To take an example from the screening form for Professionalism, a doctor might be thought to have difficulties with the following competencies:

   'Is organised, efficient and takes appropriate responsibility'
   'Deals appropriately with stress'

   The deeper features that underlie this area of performance might suggest why this might be. For example:

   - Able to admit mistakes/learn from them
   - Backs own judgment appropriately
   - Recognises own limitations and can compromise
   - Able to seek help when necessary

   We can see from this how the screening forms can be used to investigate and diagnose a problem at a competency level and also at a deeper level of performance.

4. Because RDMp areas do not stand alone but overlap with each other, the next step might be to look at problems shown up in one cluster and check for problems in associated areas. For example, Relationship & Diagnostics overlap with each other, particularly in the area of data gathering & interpretation.

   If the doctor had problems with data-gathering we could look at the **Diagnostics** screening form where we might see that the doctor had problems with the following deeper features:

   Didn't do this: Elicits necessary detail
   Did this: Fails to explore important cues/overlooks important issues

   This might prompt us to look at the screening form for **Relationship**. By completing this form, concerns might arise over the deeper features because the doctor:

   Didn't do this: Non-judgemental, shows interest and understanding, encourages contribution
   Did this: Makes assumptions, authoritarian, lacks warmth in voice/manner

   This exercise would help us to see that the data-gathering problem was not really tied in with a lack of diagnostic expertise, but was more likely to be due to a *lack of interest* in encouraging sufficient information from the patient.

5. The deeper features are shown on the screening forms, but they are an abbreviated version of what was referred to earlier in this chapter as being our 'DNA'. The full version is shown in the first chapter of each RDMp section of the book. In these short chapters, the deeper features that are particularly relevant to that section are listed and explained. Deeper features often appear in more than one section but have more impact in some areas of performance than in others. This weighting is also illustrated in the chapters.

6. The final stage is to bring these pieces together in the summary box at the bottom of the screening form and make a plan of action. We can see from the above that it is vital to take care with the diagnosis of the

problem before launching on a solution. For example, the doctor who was having problems with data-gathering would find it much harder to improve if relationship skills were not identified as being the primary problem.

The screening forms also help us to plan how best to evaluate the improvement in performance that the trainee will be working towards when the action plan is implemented.

Awareness-raising techniques

In each chapter, there are numerous boxes that are designed to expand upon the text, make connections and thereby improve insight. These boxes are of various types that ask questions, give tips and make comments about learning and about assessment. A number of competencies are thought to be particularly important and these are annotated with a 'key' symbol as mastering these can help to unlock the meaning of the domain of which they are a part.

What are the stages of learning?

So far, we've looked at ways in which we can think about the curriculum and, by using the competencies, learn to develop behaviour in order to become GPs. However, where do we start? This final model, which is based upon the patient-centred clinical method, shows how we can make use of what we already know, making it the foundation of further development. Trainees do not come into GP training as complete novices. They usually already know how to consult with patients in secondary care and this is a vital anchor point for the rest of GP specialist training. We can illustrate this idea in the following diagrams (Figures 2 & 3). The headings come from the core statement of the curriculum.

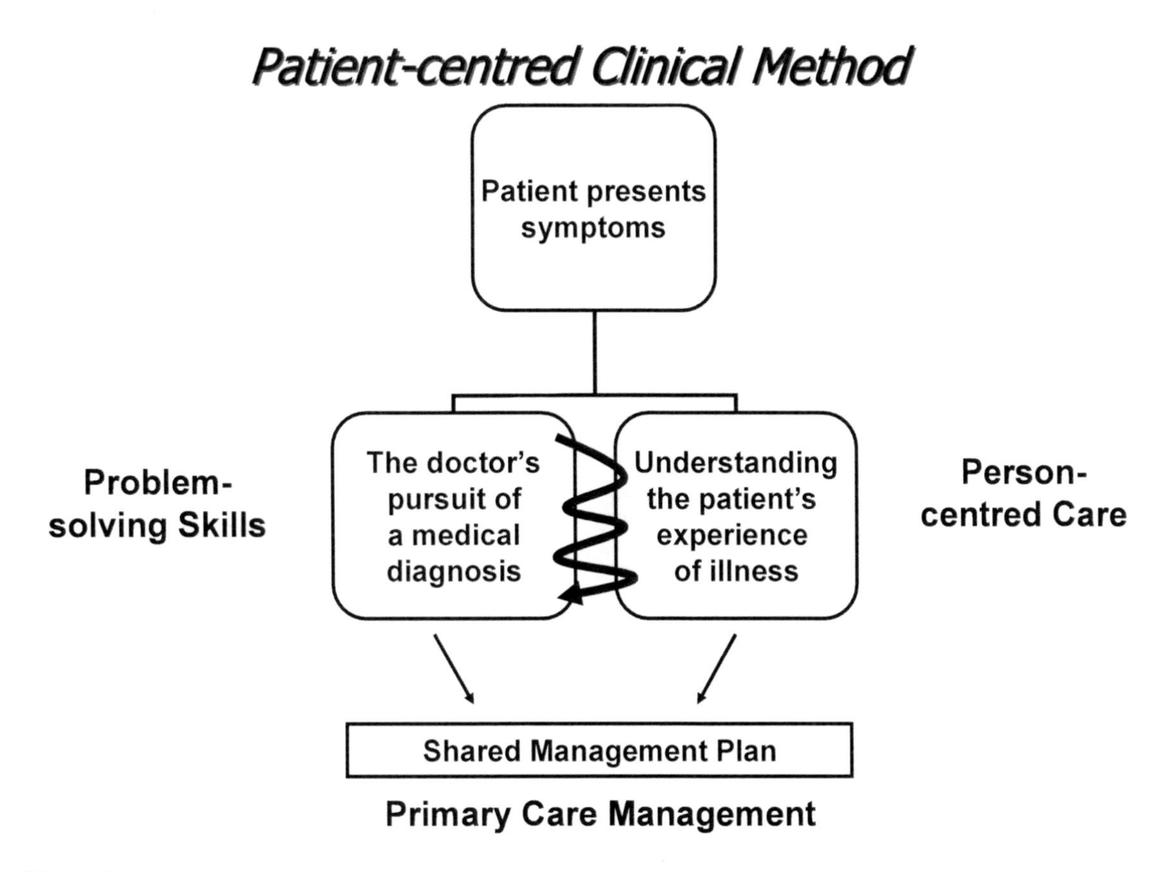

Figure 2

Figure 2 shows how the consultation begins with the patient presenting symptoms to the doctor. There then follows an attempt to understand the patient's experience of illness by exploring the patient's agenda, health beliefs & preferences. Whilst doing so, the doctor gathers information, clarifies the problem and begins to consider what management options might be appropriate. As shown by the serpentine arrow, this process involves continual dialogue between doctor and patient. As a result, doctor and patient are in a position to develop a mutually acceptable management plan that is based on a sound understanding of the nature of the problem.

Usually when doctors come into GP training, they are familiar with this model although they need time to understand the different range of illnesses that are dealt with in the community and how common symptoms can be differentiated from the early stages of more serious illnesses.

Now look at Figure 3. This shows how, with experience in primary care, each of the three boxes in figure 2, which describes skills that all doctors need irrespective of specialty, become 'enhanced' by taking on a specific primary care dimension.

Figure 3

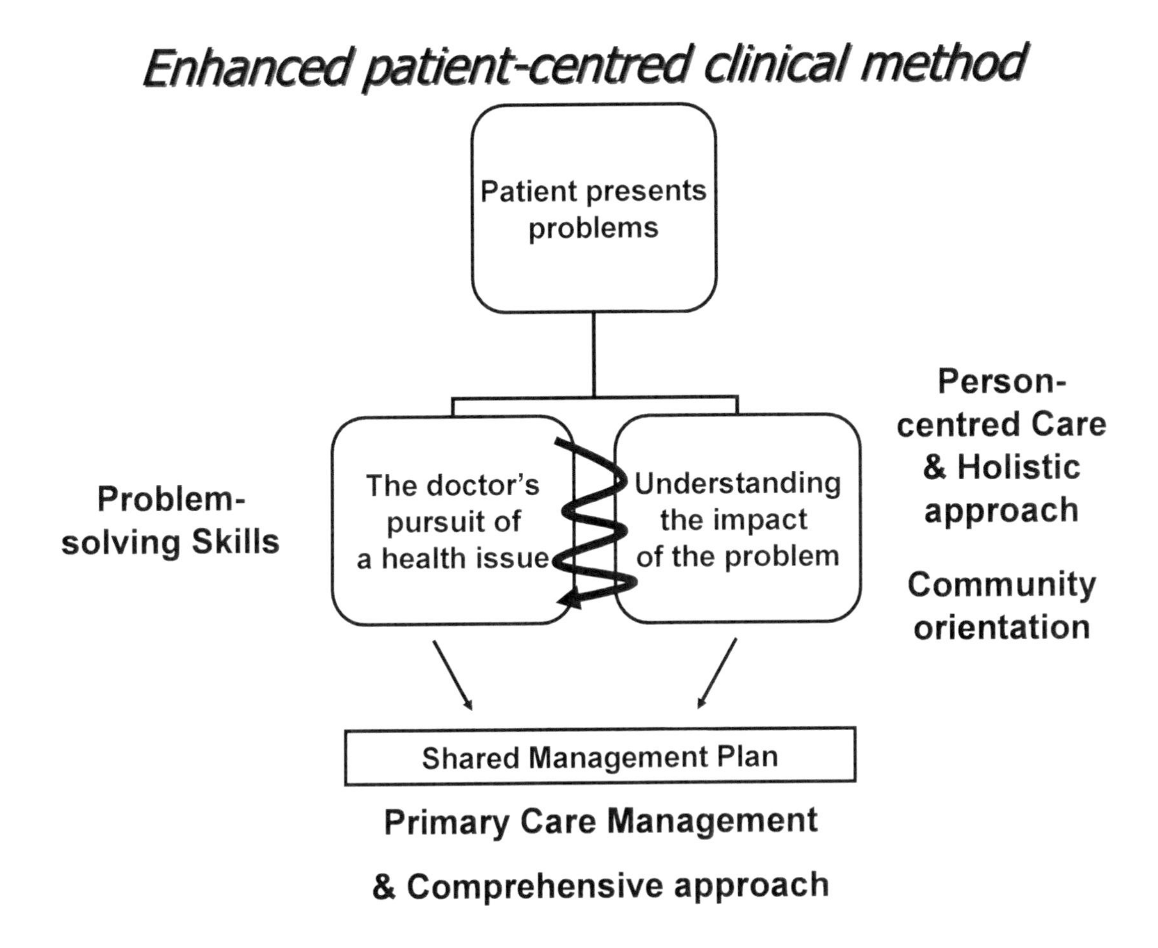

Firstly, patients do not present 'symptoms' alone, but *problems* that may or may not be the signs of disease although they may still have an impact on health. Because of this, the doctor no longer exclusively pursues a medical diagnosis, but attempts to clarify the problem and determine whether there is a health issue with which s/he can help. This problem-based approach rather than disease-based approach is a critically important feature of generalism.

Dialogue is still a central feature, but through this the doctor now searches to understand not only the patient's experience of illness but also the way in which the problem affects the patient's life and the lives of those with whom the patient is associated. What we are describing here is the 'holistic approach' to patient care.

Additionally, the doctor has an understanding of the community and is able to see how the problem might, for example, have implications for other patients in the practice and how it might be addressed by using community resources.

Through dialogue, doctor and patient can develop plans for straightforward common diseases and also for more difficult tasks such as dealing with simultaneous problems, co-morbidity and problems in evolution. The skills required to manage these challenging areas are described by the doctor's 'comprehensive approach'.

We can therefore see from this section that there is a predictable trajectory to learning that begins by practising the patient-centred clinical method with which foundation doctors are familiar and using this as a starting point, enhancing it by learning to add the primary care skills described above. Because adults learn incrementally by connecting new experiences and insights to anchor points from the past, we can see why it would be inappropriate and counter-productive to expect some of the enhanced skills described above to be present early on in GP training. This understanding can help us to tailor educational programs better and to have more realistic expectations of what can be achieved in performance terms at different stages of training.

References

Norfolk TD, Siriwardena AN. A unifying theory of general practice: relationship, diagnostics, management and professionalism (RDM-p) *Quality in Primary Care* 2009; 17, 37-47

Levenstein JH, Belle Brown J Weston WW et al (1989) Patient-centred clinical interviewing. In Communicating with medical patients (eds M Stewart and D Roter) Sage Publications, Newbury Park, CA.

Relationship

2 Relationship: Overview of the performance areas

'Relationship' is the first of the RDMp clusters and is made up of three domains from the competence framework, these being:

- Communication & consulting skills
- Practising holistically
- Working with colleagues and in teams

As the name implies, all three of these domains are concerned with human relationships, which means that if we can master the art of communicating and engaging with people, we will go a long way toward demonstrating the competencies that are described in these domains. 'Relationship' abilities are not the same as diagnostic ones, but the two are related in that 'Relationship' allows connections of trust to be made between individuals so that the diagnostic and clinical management tasks can be facilitated. Let us look at the domains in a little more detail to illustrate this point.

The first two are both dependent upon good communication with patients. Put simply, communicating well involves being interested in the patients problem, listening actively and encouraging the patients contribution, sharing ideas, explaining well and then checking what the patient has understood.

Initially, communication may focus on the problem that the patient has come with, clarifying the nature of the problem in a way that helps us to think about clinical management options. As we can become more experienced and recognise that problems in primary care are generally more complex than making a diagnosis and giving treatment, we begin to explore the problem in a broader (or holistic) context.

This broader context encompasses aspects such as the social and psychological impact of the condition on the life of the patient and the patient's family. In addition, a holistic approach takes into account the patients feelings as well as their thinking.

Exploring these facets requires certain attitudes, such as interest and understanding along with more sophisticated communication skills to probe, clarify, challenge, negotiate and so on.

The ability to develop and maintain relationships is vital for the first two domains but is also important to the third domain which concerns teamworking. In the teamworking context, our relationship skills are evident in the way we find out about the team members and their roles, the efforts we make to communicate effectively, the feedback we give team members and any other efforts we make to encourage team development.

The insights that 'Relationship' gives us helps us to see that 'teamworking' is much more than making oneself accessible or knowing about the roles and responsibilities of team members.

The deeper features are our DNA. Although few in number, they underpin all the behaviours described in the competence framework and are described in terms of knowledge, skills, attitudes and personal qualities. The behaviours being tested in the 'Relationship' section are shown in the table below, where the categories indicate the degree of weighting.

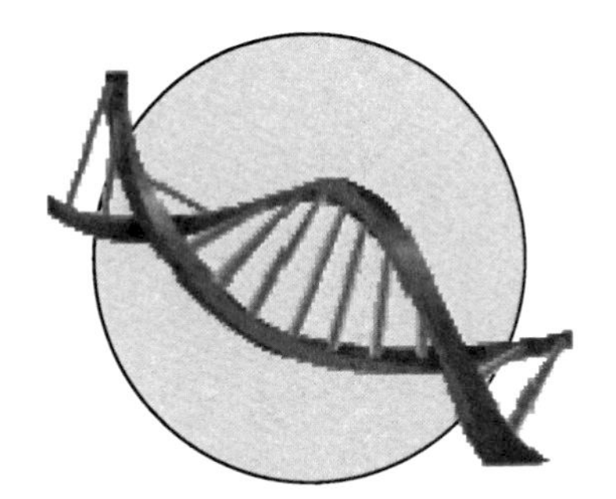

The behaviours are shown in the left-hand column. We will describe these in greater detail to clarify what they are. As you read them, use the table to cross-reference them to the domains that they underpin. This will increase your understanding and help you to develop the skills you need for each area of performance. The weighting will help you here. For example, 'working with colleagues and in teams' requires relatively little empathy and sensitivity compared to teamworking and communication skills.

If you are (or your trainee is) having a problem with performance in a domain look at the underlying deeper features for guidance on where the problem might lie and therefore which behaviours need working on.

How would we know if empathy and sensitivity were poorly developed?

Does the doctor look uninterested in what the patient is saying?

Is the doctor passive or insufficiently active in encouraging the patient?

Does the doctor appear cold, authoritarian or insensitive to feelings?

Does the atmosphere being generated seem uncomfortable?

	Communication & consulting skills	Practising holistically	Working with colleagues and in teams
Empathy & sensitivity	High	High	
Team involvement & managing others		Medium	High
Communication skills	High		Medium

Empathy and sensitivity:

- Showing interest and understanding, when responding to needs and concerns of patients and team members.
- Being open and non-judgemental.
- Taking active measures to include people in discussion and to work cooperatively with them.
- Using tone of voice and body language to indicate warmth and thereby encourage people to contribute.
- Taking steps to create a safe and trusting atmosphere through language, demeanour and behaviour.

Communication skills:

- Using patient-centred questions that encourage contribution.
- Using open questions when possible and where appropriate (for example, closed questions are appropriate for certain elements of history taking).
- Modifying approaches as required by the situation, to improve communication. For example, in the way questions are asked, explanations are given and body language used.

Team involvement and managing others:

- Communicating with team members in a non-confrontational manner.
- Listening and showing respect for other people's views.
- Negotiating and where appropriate, compromising.
- Demonstrating an even-handed approach, treating people consistently and giving constructive feedback.
- Delegating and where needed, taking the lead.

How would we know if communication was poorly developed?

Are too many closed questions used in situations where open questions would have been more fruitful?

Does the doctor fail to adapt their verbal / nonverbal communication in line with what the patient or colleague needs?

How would you know if team involvement was poorly developed?

Does the doctor show favouritism toward some colleagues compared to others?

Is the doctor confrontational or unhelpfully critical?

Does the doctor fail to take account of other people's views and concerns?

Does the doctor fail to take action when concerns are expressed about his/her skills?

3 Relationship: Communication and consultation skills

This area of performance is about communication with patients and the use of recognised consultation techniques.

Needs Further Development	Competent for licensing	Excellent	
Develops a working relationship with the patient, but one in which the problem rather than the person is the focus.	Explores the patient's agenda, health beliefs and preferences. Elicits psychological and social information to place the patient's problem in context.	Incorporates the patient's perspective and context when negotiating the management plan.	**1**

This first progression illustrates how we move from:

A problem-centred consulting approach, through

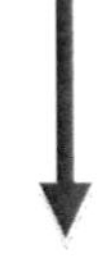

Regular efforts to understand the patient's perspective and the impact of the patient's problem on their lives

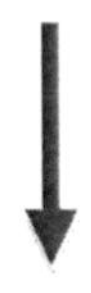

Developing management plans that reflect this understanding

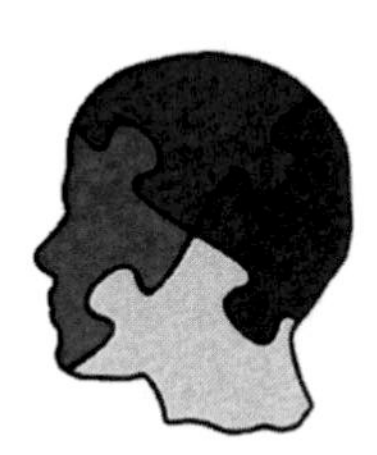

Joined up?
See p14

Looking at each of the word pictures in turn:

Develops a working relationship with the patient, but one in which the problem rather than the person is the focus.

Doctors who demonstrate this level of competence develop a working (or functional) relationship with the patient that can achieve results but does not necessarily reflect any depth of relationship between doctor and patient. Because the relationship element is not well-developed, it is unlikely that the patient's problems are understood by the doctor in the context of the patient's life or that management plans are particularly sophisticated.

Question

If we think about patient factors rather than our own communication skills, in what situations might it be difficult to establish rapport with the patient?

Normally, rapport is fairly straightforward to establish with most patients. However, in some situations it can be tricky. For example, there may be patients who have permanent communication difficulties such as those who have had a stroke or who have learning disabilities. The challenge here is for us to maintain a patient-centred approach even when communication involves carers and other intermediaries.

Sometimes, there may be a combination of factors that impede communication. For example, patients with drug & alcohol misuse problems could have communication problems because of their condition, and might be met with negative emotions (through our prejudice, fear etc) that make rapport even more difficult to achieve. Similarly, patients with mental health problems, learning difficulties and those from other cultures may be more challenging to establish rapport with.

Why is this word picture labelled NFD (needs further development)? This is because to achieve the next step (competent), we have to focus on the patient rather than simply the problem. In most circumstances, this should be possible although sometimes, such as when the patient has an acute or emergency problem, this may not be possible or even appropriate. Arguably, in these circumstances we could demonstrate patient-centredness by trying to understand the patient's thoughts and preferences through the relatives.

Explores the patient's agenda, health beliefs and preferences.

This behaviour is felt by educators to be particularly important.

Assessor's corner: being patient-centred

Does the trainee take an interest in the patient and recognise that they are dealing with a person rather than a problem?

Sometimes, trainees may misunderstand patient-centredness, believing this to mean that they should simply accede to the patient's wishes. Once again, the patient, as a person, has not really being taken account of and the doctor is simply being *reactive* rather than responsive.

The key skill here is to 'explore', in other words not to passively accept what is offered by the patient, but probe further until we are happy that we have a good understanding of the patient's ideas concerns and expectations about the problem. All patients have thoughts, but many need help with expressing and clarifying these. For example, men may be less articulate about their health compared with women and some may be apologetic ('I didn't want to come, but my partner made me'). Don't let this fool you as such patients are usually no less concerned about their health than the average person, sometimes more so!

Exploring the patient's thoughts requires us to put patients at their ease, particularly if, as with sexual health or bowel conditions, the patient might find such discussion embarrassing. Sometimes, 'exploring' may mean that we have to challenge a patient's thoughts, for example whether or not they are ready to quit smoking.

Patients and their families not only have thoughts about the problems, but also about what they expect from the practice and the health service more generally. Exploring these thoughts (e.g. 'what did you hope that we might do about this problem?') is not only good consulting practice, but can help us to tailor the management plan more appropriately to the patient's needs and thereby reduce dissatisfaction with the service.

Elicits psychological and social information to place the patient's problem in context.

The object here is to understand whether, how and to what degree a problem is having an impact on the life of the patient. We might explore to see if a psychological problem is present as this often coexists with more significant physical problems and may not be recognised or admitted by the patient. The fact that psychological problems can lead to physical disease is often overlooked, particularly in those with enduring mental illness. What does 'social impact' mean? It may involve relationships, the workplace and especially for younger patients, education.

Every problem has the capacity to have a wider impact both in the patient and in those associated with him or her. Sometimes, such an impact might be anticipated, for example with patients who have visual difficulties or patients with skin problems that cause disfigurement. Sometimes, the impact may not be obvious or may not be mentioned to us, as a result of which it may not be considered. For example, domestic violence in women and physical abuse of the elderly are prevalent but are easily overlooked.

Incorporates the patient's perspective and context when negotiating the management plan.

Having elicited the information above, at the 'excellent' end of the scale this competence is achieved when the management plan is discussed and developed by explicitly incorporating the patient's perspective and context. The classification of 'excellent' is because negotiation can involve challenge and conflict and is therefore a difficult area of communication.

What do the words perspective and context mean in practice? For example, the patient's perspective may determine whether a drug or non-drug approach is chosen or whether (when appropriate) they wish to live with a problem rather than be referred and so on.

The patient's context may include the nature of their illness and its interaction with other conditions from which they suffer, the employer's attitude to sickness absence, whether the patient has dependents, the availability of help and so on. Any of these could have an impact upon a proposed management plan.

There is considerable overlap between this section and 'practising holistically'. The difference is that this section is concerned with the communication skills used to achieve a holistic objective, whereas 'practising holistically' concentrates on the use made of holistic information.

Computers and communication

The consulting room computer is a relatively recent but significant threat to establishing and maintaining a relationship with the patient. Look at yourself on video and ask yourself if you are becoming too *'computer-centred'*.

Sometimes, repositioning the computer can help to reduce the time spent looking away or even worse, turning away, from the patient. Involving the patient in the use of the computer is another way of keeping attention focused on the patient and their problem.

Assessor's corner: putting the problem in context

Does the trainee elicit psychosocial information when history taking? Look for a disparity between what the trainee says that they would do (e.g. in CbD) and what they actually do in COT.

In case-discussion, try to discuss psychosocial issues. If they haven't been asked about by the trainee, no meaningful discussion can take place.

Needs Further Development	Competent for licensing	Excellent
Produces management plans that are appropriate to the patient's problem.	Works in partnership with the patient, negotiating a mutually acceptable plan that respects the patient's agenda and preference for involvement.	Whenever possible, adopts plans that respect the patient's autonomy.

2

Incorporating the patient's perspective: what is the evidence?

This competence centres on negotiation and the doctor's willingness to modify management plans. Watch a consultation: are the patient's preferences discussed?

Are initial ideas about the plan changed or tailored in the light of the patient's preferences.

This second progression illustrates how we move from:

Producing a plan that seems appropriate to the problem, but doing so without significant patient involvement

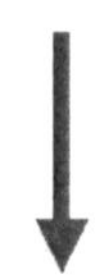

Engaging in dialogue that results in a negotiated plan

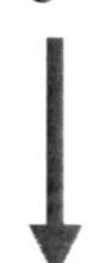

Ensuring that plans are, wherever possible, patient-centred

Looking at each of the word pictures in turn:

Produces management plans that are appropriate to the patient's problem.

This behaviour is usually straightforward, although we need to remember that 'problems' are not always diseases. The major emphasis, however, is on clinical care.

Sometimes, an appropriate management plan may not be immediately obvious. This may mean that we have to wait and review the patient within a specified time frame to see how the condition evolves. Occasionally it may mean that we have to admit that no more intervention can be offered, for example when curative options are exhausted. However, this should not be seen as being a bleak or hopeless outcome as there are always other options. As has been said, doctors should 'cure sometimes, palliate often and comfort always'.

What we need to remember is that this behaviour lies in the *communication* domain rather than pure clinical management which means that to demonstrate it, we have to show that we have developed a sufficiently good relationship to recommend an appropriate management plan, particularly through the desire to engage and the ability to listen attentively. At this level of achievement, we are not yet 'competent' because we are not yet working in partnership.

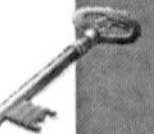

Works in partnership with the patient, negotiating a mutually acceptable plan that respects the patient's agenda and preference for involvement.

This competence is felt by many educators to be the most important in the communication skills domain.

The key competence here is our ability to adopt a partnership mindset, characterised by the desire to work as joint experts in which we contribute medical expertise and the patient contributes expertise about themselves to the management plan. Put another way, doctors bring medical evidence and patients bring the 'evidence' of their values and preferences . Additionally, doctors need to have the skills to negotiate a plan that respects the patient's viewpoint but also exemplifies good clinical management.

Sometimes, perhaps for personal or cultural reasons or because of physical frailty, patients may prefer not to be involved in developing the plan and may then abdicate responsibility to ourselves. As long as we have genuinely tried to involve the patient, rather than assumed that they are reluctant to engage, we will have demonstrated the communication skill that this competency requires.

Of course, a plan may *appear* to be negotiated, but may not be followed by the patient. If this happens more frequently than we would anticipate, we might ask ourselves whether we are truly negotiating and whether we really elicit the patient's preferences before making our own preferences known.

Whenever possible, adopts plans that respect the patient's autonomy.

The opportunity for this may sometimes be limited, for example if the patient has insufficient mental capacity either through acute illness or long-term problems such as learning disability. We may need to involve other people who can speak on the patient's behalf and sometimes this can cause a conflict of views between parties who each believe that they are acting in the patient's best interest. Autonomy may be tailored as the patient develops. For example, young children may have little autonomy but older children and adolescents are capable of giving informed consent within certain parameters, as laid out in guidelines such as Gillick or Fraser competence.

Ask yourself: How often do you try talking to children directly, rather than through adults?

Question: How might empowering the patient be helpful when negotiating a management plan?

Other management approaches require doctors to empower their patients, for example to adopt self-treatment and coping strategies for relatively minor conditions like hay fever, but more importantly for significant / chronic conditions like asthma where the day-to-day management is best when under the patient's control.

Assessor's corner: negotiating a plan

Look closely at COT. Does the doctor provide a legitimate range of management options, explaining the pros and cons of each approach? Does the doctor avoid well-meaning dictatorship, in which they simply choose on behalf of the patient?

Assessor's corner: respecting the patient's autonomy

Does the trainee facilitate autonomy by explaining well and providing information about the implications of the available choices? Does the trainee override the patient or criticise their preference?

Needs Further Development	Competent for licensing	Excellent	
Provides explanations that are relevant and understandable to the patient, using appropriate language.	Explores the patient's understanding of what has taken place.	Uses a variety of communication techniques and materials to adapt explanations to the needs of the patient.	3

This third progression illustrates how we move from:

Providing explanations that are capable of being understood by the patient

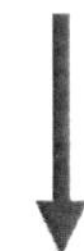

Checking what the patient has understood and whether this understanding is correct

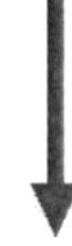

When communication is more challenging, using techniques to make sure that the messages are understood

Looking at each of the word pictures in turn:

Provides explanations that are relevant and understandable to the patient, using appropriate language

Good explanations rarely, unless talking to other health professionals, use technical language. The ability to phrase in plain English, using colloquial language when appropriate and (even better) use the patient's preferred phrases, not only helps us to make good explanations but greatly increases the chance that the explanation will be properly understood - and believed. All patients deserve explanations, even when their capacity to understand is poor, for example in children and those with intellectual impairments. Good GPs will do their best to involve the patient and tailor explanations so that what they say is useful and does not cause avoidable distress. Sometimes this can simply be to inform patients that a full explanation is being given to someone they trust such as a parent or carer.

Explanations help patients to make choices. One of the most challenging areas is when we are required to explain risk, for example the risk of cardiovascular events or the risk of complications from obesity and diabetes. Here, language may not be enough on its own and pictorial illustrations of risk may be needed to clarify and reinforce the message.

Good explanation is not just part of good communicating. By explaining well, better choices can be made, concordance can be improved and the risk to patient safety that might result from misunderstandings can be reduced. Also, a careful choice of words can help patients to have a more positive approach to improvement. For example, patients with rheumatic disorders may respond better to being told about 'wear and repair' than about 'disintegrating joints'.

Assessor's corner: exploring the patient's understanding

It may be obvious from COT whether or not the trainee asks what the patient has understood. More subtly, does the trainee follow-up on non-verbal cues that indicate that the patient may be confused, unsure or disbelieving?

Explores the patient's understanding of what has taken place.

Explanations may seem to be going well, especially when the patient gives non-verbal cues such as smiling and nodding at us when we speak. However, they may simply be being polite! Studies show that patients recall little of what is said and therefore it is not surprising that they may misunderstand some of the detail, for example how often tablets are to be taken or when their condition should be reviewed. Sometimes, they may have entirely misunderstood the *substance* of the explanation. For instance, despite our best efforts at explaining, patients may believe themselves to be diabetic when they have glycosuria but a normal fasting sugar.

Uses a variety of communication techniques and materials to adapt explanations to the needs of the patient.

This is a higher level competence because the ability to adapt in a variety of ways comes from experience of patient needs and from proficiency with consulting skills. Examples include commonplace activities such as communicating effectively with patients who have hearing impairment, for example by remembering to face the patient and speak clearly to let them lip-read. Sometimes, diagrams and drawings may be needed and Internet-based information is increasingly useful either during the consultation or as homework. Depending on the nature of the local population, patients may require interpreters. Here, part of the communication challenge for us is to remain patient-focused by looking at and talking to the patient rather than to the third party.

Assessor's corner: adapting explanations

Look closely at COT. Does the trainee use a 'one size fits all' approach? Does s/he vary explanations, for example tailoring them to the needs of different types of patients (age, gender, ethnic groups etc)?

Rather than adapt the explanation, does the trainee appear frustrated or angry if the patient appears not to understand?

We mentioned autonomy in the previous section and the heart of respecting the patient's autonomy is to provide sufficient information and explanation in a form that the patient understands. To do this, we will need to tailor our language, speak clearly and so on, but we may also need to back this up with communication aids like diagrams and leaflets as described in this section.

Providing explanations is not the sole responsibility of the GP. We should encourage questioning by the patient and encourage the patient, their carer and family to access further information and use patient support groups when appropriate.

Needs Further Development	Competent for licensing	Excellent
Achieves the tasks of the consultation but uses a rigid approach.	Flexibly and efficiently achieves consultation tasks, responding to the consultation preferences of the patient.	Appropriately uses advanced consultation skills such as confrontation or catharsis to achieve better patient outcomes.

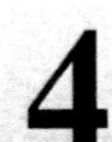

This fourth progression illustrates how we move from:

An inexpert approach to consulting, which at this basic level can look like a process of consulting 'by numbers'. For example, we may go through every consultation in a formulaic manner, irrespective of the nature of the problem or the personality of the patient.

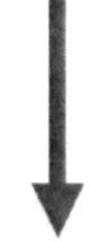

A competent and fluid approach in which consultation tasks may be performed in a variety of sequences according to the circumstances rather than in a predetermined order. For example, we may listen, take some history, explore some management options and then come back to further history taking, doing so without disturbing the flow of the dialogue.

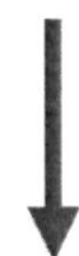

We not only have a fluid technique but, when the situation demands, may use special communication skills. For example when we have hit an impasse in dealing with the problem we may use interventions such as helping the patient to release emotional tension (catharsis) and encouraging the patient to problem-solve through reflection and self-discovery (catalysis).

Looking at each of the word pictures in turn:

Achieves the tasks of the consultation but uses a rigid approach.

Doctors who perform at this level are conversant with basic skills. They 'tick the boxes' but lack flexibility and fluency. If consulting *skills* are basic, then the consultation *outcomes* are likely to reflect this. It is therefore less likely that difficult situations such as dealing with multiple problems and hidden agendas will be tackled well.

Flexibly and efficiently achieves consultation tasks, responding to the consultation preferences of the patient.

Different patients require different approaches. This may be obvious when there is a language barrier. Less obviously, we may have to tailor our consultation approach to the needs of groups such as children, pregnant women, the elderly or the housebound. Culture also makes a difference. For example, in some cultures there is less willingness to accept the Western model of shared decision-making and patients may prefer what we would call a 'doctor-centred' consultation model. However, we should take care not to *assume* that this is the case as it is increasingly rare for patients from any culture to unquestioningly accept our advice in the way they did a generation ago.

Appropriately uses advanced consultation skills such as confrontation or catharsis to achieve better patient outcomes.

At the excellent end of the scale, we help patients to become better-able to share in decision-making by encouraging them to question more, understand the issues better, become more aware of their motivating factors and to be more accountable for keeping their side of the management-plan bargain. This not only requires the patient's trust, usually built upon the bedrock of an existing relationship, but also requires advanced communication skills that include the abilities to challenge, question, inform and negotiate.

The skills involved in consulting with patients can help greatly with other aspects of medical practice. As we will see later, they can assist us to communicate with teams, groups and organisations in order to improve services and achieve change.

Looking to the future, when all doctors will have some role in teaching, there are striking similarities between consulting skills and the skills required for effective teaching, in particular active listening, questioning and summarising to help reach a shared understanding of the problem or issue that needs to be addressed. Maybe this should make us think of our consultations as being *learning* opportunities and voyages of discovery? Not always easy last thing on a Friday afternoon!

Learning more advanced consulting skills

Watch more experienced doctors consult and look to see how they jump about with consultation tasks rather than pursue them in a linear fashion. In particular, look out for patient cues (e.g. remarks that are dropped or facial expressions).

These are often significant and good consulters will pick up on them and come back to them, weaving them in to the consultation later on.

Try to make notes when you sit in on consultations, perhaps using the COT schedule so that you can learn to recognise these more advanced skills and see what they can achieve.

What are the deeper features that underpin communication?

This is a good time to go back to the deeper features. Look closely at those listed under empathy & sensitivity and communication skills.

Ask someone more experienced to give you some feedback on these. Are there any that you feel are weaknesses for you? How would you work on them?

4 Relationship: Practising holistically

This performance area is about the ability of doctors to operate in physical, psychological, socio-economic and cultural dimensions, taking into account feelings as well as thoughts.

Holism may sound like a relatively abstract concept, but it embodies the broader mindset that characterises good GPs and the way in which they see problems and their effects as part of a bigger picture. *Why is this important?* It is because health has many dimensions and is affected by a variety of factors beyond the simple causes of disease. For example, holism means recognising that what the patient thinks and feels about an illness can strongly influence the degree to which they suffer *and* the rapidity with which they recover. Also, holism means recognising that the factors that aid recovery are much broader than the therapies available through traditional Medicine and include psychological approaches, social interventions, complementary medicine and so on.

A holistic approach is therefore not some form of a abstract GP creed, but has real practical significance, especially when problems are complex and treatment approaches are not clear-cut.

Holism has a number of meanings, but to illustrate its range and depth, here is a definition that we commonly use:

Holism is defined as 'caring for the whole person in the context of the person's values, his family beliefs, their family system and their culture in the larger community and considering a range of therapies based on the evidence of their benefits and cost'

This shows us that Holism, one of the core values of general practice, is very strongly linked to patient-centredness which is another core value.

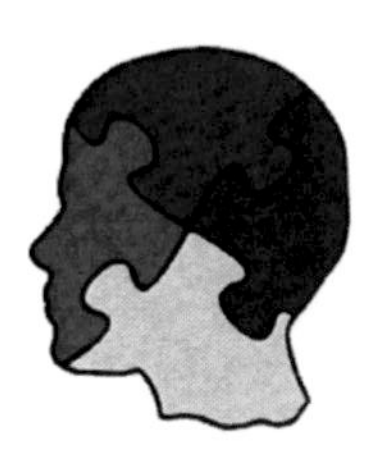

Joined up?
See p14

Holism is often condensed to the shorthand of 'integrating physical, psychological and social components of health problems', the so-called bio-psycho-social model of illness. Practising holistically means not only having a holistic mindset, but also knowing how to translate this understanding into practical measures that improve the patient's health. For example, holistic practitioners will offer a wider range of options than simply medical ones (as mentioned above) and will also use other sources of help for the patient than just themselves.

Not surprisingly, when we look at the DNA, our deeper features, to practise holistically we need to show a good deal of empathy and sensitivity. This makes sense, because these attributes help us to be open and non-judgemental. Without them we cannot learn to value such things as the other approaches to health

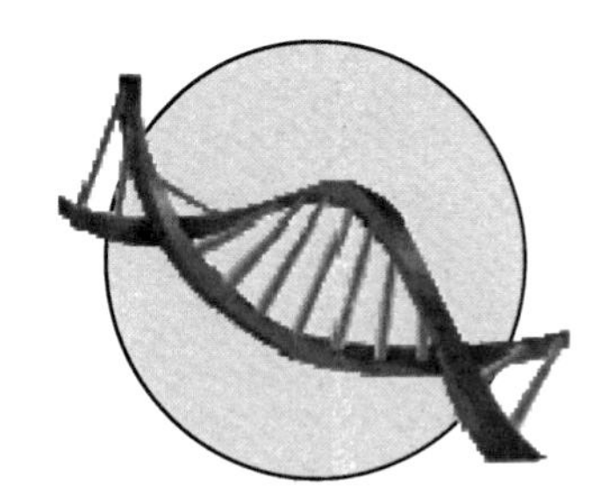

care, the patient's thoughts and beliefs and the importance of how the problem is affecting the patient's life.

The thread of empathy and sensitivity also explains why 'practising holistically' is strongly related to communication and consulting skills, where as we have seen in the DNA box on page 24, it is also of great importance.

The performance area of practising holistically is described in three major themes or indicator progressions, which we will now look at in detail.

Needs Further Development	Competent for licensing	Excellent
Enquires into both physical and psychological aspects of the patient's problem.	Demonstrates understanding of the patient in relation to their socio-economic and cultural background.	Uses this understanding to inform discussion and to generate practical suggestions for patient management.

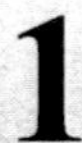

Tip

This section overlaps with the first indicator progression statement in the 'communication & consultation skills' performance area.

See page 27

This first progression illustrates how we move from:

Asking about physical and psychological aspects of the patient's problem. This may not sound much, but without this step, we are poorly equipped to understand the *effect* of the problem.

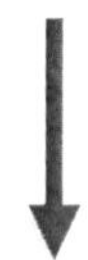

Not only asking about, but also demonstrating that we understand the relationship between the patient and elements of their social, occupational and cultural background

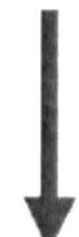

Actively making use of this new understanding by discussing how the management plan can be tailored to take account of these factors.

Looking at each of the word pictures in turn:

Enquires into both physical and psychological aspects of the patient's problem.

This indicator is the first step in looking in a more holistic way at the patient's problem.

In any illness, physical and psychological factors may coexist. Physical illnesses have psychological sequelae and vice versa. For example, we often see psychosomatic symptoms manifest themselves as musculoskeletal problems, and we also know that musculoskeletal problems often have an important psychological component such as low mood.

Some physical symptoms, for example the so-called 'functional disorders' may be manifestations of psychological distress. These disorders include irritable bowel syndrome, non-ulcer dyspepsia and abdominal pain in children. Likewise, certain ENT symptoms such as globus may be the presentation of psychological problems, in this case anxiety.

This physical/psychological duality also manifests itself in the way patients choose to talk about, understand or accept (or not) their condition, with some patients experiencing the problem in physical terms and others in psychological (including emotional) ways.

Demonstrates understanding of the patient in relation to their socio-economic and cultural background.

Many educators consider this to be the most important competence in the whole performance area.

One of the challenges and joys of general practice is learning how people understand their health in relation to their world. Understanding British people means, in our multicultural society, understanding how people from diverse backgrounds think about health and illness, both how they are caused and how doctors can help. Overcoming personal resistance and prejudice in order to achieve this understanding is the starting point for learning to value the differences between people. We will revisit this point when we consider diversity on page 194.

Let's be more specific about how diversity and holism are linked. Social and cultural diversity particularly about diet, nutrition, gastrointestinal function and mental health really affects the health beliefs that patients have. To give two examples, some cultures regard what we would call 'hallucinations' as being normal experiences. Others, particularly from tropical countries, may understandably regard fever as being indicative of possibly fatal disease, rather than being a self-limiting 'minor' illness. Our 'empathy and sensitivity' deeper features are once again important here because if we do not have an open and non-judgemental approach, we can easily misunderstand or worse still, misdiagnose the patient. Thus in the examples just given, patients with hallucinations may be misdiagnosed as psychotic and those with viral illnesses as being neurotic.

Culture may affect how people think, but it also has a number of practical consequences. For example, culture may strongly influence naming systems, rites of passage rituals such as circumcision, personal ethics, expectations in terminal illness and death rituals. Culture is a holistic matter and as we can appreciate, it could have a powerful influence on how to best manage the patient.

Developing a holistic mindset

Even if you think your consultation has been one-dimensional, try to learn about the psychosocial dimension of the patient's problem by using computer codes and search facilities to explore and integrate the physical, psychological and social components that may appear in the records.

For example, what other physical, psychological or social problems are present?

Could these affect or be affected by the current problem? For instance, what about employment; could this be a factor?

Assessor's corner

Does the doctor ignore cues? The COT has a section on enquiring into psychological and social factors. Look at the trainee's scores in this area. If they remain persistently low, further action may be needed.

This might include looking at video consultations, stopping and starting the tape and asking 'what might the patient be thinking at this point?' or 'what other questions would you ask to explore psychological and social issues that might be relevant here?'

Holism does not just apply to cultures that are different from the indigenous one. The culture of British society itself has a profound effect on how people view their illness. For instance, British people are on the whole expected to be stoical. Also, British society (as with all societies) stigmatises some people and some behaviours. Therefore, people who smoke or who are obese are singled out in the media for particular scorn. Increasingly, doctors are at the sharp end of implementing government policy for example with smoking cessation and the medicalisation of obesity. Having a holistic mindset means that we should become aware of the potential effects of stigmatisation and take steps to reduce these.

Understanding patients also means understanding the ways in which they view the world. Unlike doctors, who are trained to look at health in (principally) scientific ways, patients don't usually take this approach, but seek to understand health in relation to their personal and family values and beliefs. Therefore, patients may voice their beliefs by saying, for instance, that some things happen because they are 'in the family', that taking tablets is 'not how I was brought up', that 'my father never took a day off work' or that 'uncle Fred smoked every day of his life and lived to 90'.

These values and beliefs are deep-seated and powerful. Having a holistic mindset means that we seek them out, respect them and wherever possible make constructive use of them. If we don't, our efforts might be misdirected and patient care might become frustrating for reasons that we don't immediately understand or respect.

Connecting holism with diversity in your community

You may wish, or need, to learn about how different cultural groups in your patient community approach health and illness. You can learn about this from patients directly, from community leaders and from books.

Ask your colleagues how they have practised holistically with these groups. For example, how have they modified their diagnostic and treatment approaches as a consequence of their cultural awareness?

Uses this understanding to inform discussion and to generate practical suggestions for patient management.

Once we understand the practical importance of holism, we are more likely to help the patient by discussing the problem more widely, using this to generate a broader range of practical options than we would otherwise have considered.

'Discussing more widely' means enabling the patient to disclose the factors that they think influence the problem and how it might be resolved, without fear of being embarrassed or ridiculed. Once we see for ourselves that holism leads to more effective management plans, it quickly becomes a central part of the way we work rather than an optional add-on.

Assessor's corner

To understand holism, the doctor should be open-minded and non-judgemental. There may be positive evidence of this.

Alternatively, there may be evidence that the doctor does *not* have this mindset. For example, does s/he display prejudice either in face-to-face patient contact or in discussions outside the consultation?

Needs Further Development	Competent for licensing	Excellent
Recognises the impact of the problem on the patient.	Additionally, recognises the impact of the problem on the patient's family/ carers.	Recognises and shows understanding of the limits of the doctor's ability to intervene in the holistic care of the patient.

2

This second progression illustrates how we move from:

Recognising that the problem does not exist in isolation, but becomes significant because of a negative effect on the patient's life.

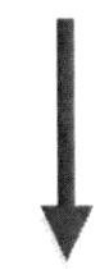

Recognising that patients rarely live in isolation. Problems that affect them will also have an effect on those that care for or about them, with possible wider health consequences that we have to consider as part of our holistic approach.

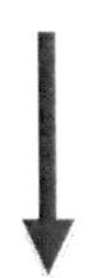

Demonstrating that although we can offer practical help and support with the narrow problem, our ability to influence the wider context, even when this is understood, is limited.

Insight from the curriculum

The curriculum says that 'blindness separates people from things. Deafness separates people from people'. How does this help you to understand the holistic approach?

Recognises the impact of the problem on the patient.

We may think that the impact of a problem is obvious, but sometimes this is an assumption. To be a good holistic practitioner, it is important not to assume but to clarify, as new and possibly important insights are often there to be gained if we are interested enough to enquire.

We should ask about the psychosocial impact of problems as this may influence the management options that are discussed and the anticipatory care that is given. For example, long-term problems frequently lead to an increased risk of depression, relationship problems, restrictions on employment and therefore on income. Knowing this will help us to (for example) keep a close eye on the patient's mood or better still, suggest ways in which problems like depression can be anticipated and averted.

Assessor's corner

From COT, is it apparent that the trainee is either attending to cues or missing important ones, for example concerning the patient's home or work concerns?

When discussing cases, can you build up a good picture of the patient's background from the information gleaned by the trainee?

Do you know in what way the problem is affecting the patient's life? If not, holistic enquiry may be missing.

Additionally, recognises the impact of the problem on the patient's family/carers.

Following on, the patient's problem may have devastating consequences for his or her dependants. For example, the children of substance misusers are particularly vulnerable and may end up becoming carers for their own parents.

Health problems in the parents, particularly mental health issues, may lead to physical problems and to behavioural problems such as enuresis and school refusal in the children. These connections can be made if we use the holistic approach and ask about the wider effects of the parent's problem.

Assessor's corner

What other forms of help does the trainee enlist in managing the patient's problem?

Are these people/resources appropriate? How is this explained to the patient?

Parents with special needs: an example of holism

In the section on 'services to young people', the curriculum describes the need to:

'Recognise the importance of supporting parents who have special needs'

Think about the needs of children of parents with substance misuse, mental health or domestic violence problems or severe chronic or short term conditions which affect their capacity to parent their children. Some children may need referral for multi-agency assessment and support services.

This may include referral to the health visitor for a comprehensive family needs- assessment in order to understand and address the impact of the parent's needs on the children's health and development.

How else could you support these children?

Recognises and shows understanding of the limits of the doctor's ability to intervene in the holistic care of the patient.

There are always limits to our ability to intervene, and recognising these is important in determining where to stop before more harm than good is caused. Of course, this applies to all medical interventions, but with the holistic dimension (unlike prescribing, for example) we may be relatively ignorant of what can realistically be achieved.

In addition, when practising holistically we are often delving into sensitive matters and there is therefore the potential for harm. For example, a common holistic approach is to involve the family. This can be valuable but the family will have their own views and maybe their own axe to grind so it is important that we proceed sensitively, wherever possible by involving the patient.

Holism and preventative care

Family members may develop health issues that have their roots in the patient's problem. Quite often, these can be predicted. For example, we might anticipate that a patient with erectile dysfunction could develop relationship or mental health difficulties (and indeed, vice versa). These effects can be discussed before they happen and in this way, averted or minimised.

Assessor's corner

Does the trainee recognise the effect of the patient's problem on others, especially on those that the patient is dependent upon? This applies particularly to children and the elderly. To help develop this skill, trainees could spend time with others involved in holistic care such as health visitors and counsellors who can illustrate how problems have much wider effects on the patient's life.

Likewise, taking responsibility for a palliative care patient or a patient with debilitating illness such as MS can help trainees to understand the impact that some health issues have beyond the physical dimension.

Needs Further Development	Competent for licensing	Excellent
Uses him/herself as the sole means of supporting the patient.	Utilises appropriate support agencies (including primary health care team members) targeted to the needs of the patient.	Organises appropriate support for the patient's family and carers.

3

This third progression illustrates how we move from:

A plan in which we provide help and follow-up in relative isolation of others who could help, such as the team.

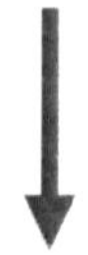

A more sophisticated approach in which the roles & abilities of team members and others such as family members are also made use of to manage the problem & support the patient.

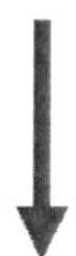

An approach in which we not only consider the impact of the problem on the patient, but also on the family and carers. As a result of this, the latter are supported along with the patient.

Holism and help

Why might a doctor use him/herself as the sole means of support?

What benefits might a patient derive from having more than one healthcare practitioner involved in the management of the problem?

Looking at each of the word pictures in turn:

Uses him/herself as the sole means of supporting the patient

It is natural to build the plan around the help that we, personally, can offer. This may come from a desire to offer personal support and this commitment is usually valued greatly by the patient.

However, such an approach is unsustainable as the patient cannot be supported long-term by one doctor. In addition, such an approach is unlikely to provide the optimum care for the patient because it doesn't encourage the use of other people and agencies who have expertise that might help the patient.

We might use ourselves as the sole means of support for a number of reasons, which we will now explore.

Occasionally, we feel it is our duty to do so perhaps because we interpret continuity of care as meaning a personal long-term commitment. This is rare nowadays as most doctors tailor their personal commitment for example by overseeing the patient's healthcare, managing some problems (such as chronic diseases) in partnership with other team members and others, such as mild depression, mostly on their own.

Sometimes, we work single-handedly because we are *unaware* of other appropriate forms of help both within the practice and without. This can happen if we don't know what's available or don't know (perhaps because we don't explore enough) what the patient needs. Rarely, the patient may be 'forbidden' from seeing another doctor perhaps because we have something to gain from dependency or because we don't wish our management to be exposed to an independent opinion or to external scrutiny.

These factors apply to all of us at some time in our career. Think carefully (and honestly) about which of these factors apply to you and what if anything you need to do to modify your approach.

Of course, we may end up being pretty much the sole form of support (or at least, feeling like it!) because of patient choice. Part of our role is to discourage dependency, where this is unhelpful, by being alert to it and by educating patients so that they understand the value of having others involved.

Holism and dependency

How would you achieve a balance between providing continuity of care and avoiding the pitfalls of dependency? What would you say to the patient?

Utilises appropriate support agencies (including primary health care team members) targeted to the needs of the patient.

Support agencies in primary & secondary care are widespread and the problem is more often with knowing what is available, accessible and how it is best used. 'Targeting' also depends upon knowing the patient's needs and this in turn requires good communication skills to identify the patient's health beliefs and expectations.

Targeting can be improved by discussing with the patient what the various possible agencies have to offer, thereby facilitating an informed choice.

'Support agencies' could also be said to include the most important support of all, i.e. the family and social network. With careful handling so that the patient understands and agrees to the involvement of other people, it can be immensely helpful to hear the perspective of others who know the patient and then work with them to provide support.

Bear in mind that sometimes the patient is simply the lightning rod for more deep-seated problems, and this can become apparent when other people are brought in to discuss the problem. For example, behavioural problems in a child are likely to suggest problems in the family or at school.

The quality of other forms of help

How would you get to know the quality of what an 'agency' such as a hospital department or a community resource has to offer? Who would you ask and what outcome measures would you look for?

Supporting the supporters

- How would you identify the carers of infirm patients?
- Having identified carers in the patient community, what issues would you discuss with them?
- What forms of help can you provide carers?
- What would you do if the carer was not one of your patients?

Organises appropriate support for the patient's family and carers.

This competence represents a very high level of holistic care, because to achieve this we must identify who else beyond the patient might be affected by the problem, whether they need to be supported and if so in what way.

One way of approaching this is to think of ourselves as constructing scaffolding around the patient to provide integrated support. The patient's family and carers would perhaps be the most important part of that support in day-to-day life and we have a role in helping them to fulfil that function.

We also have a role in identifying the forms of help that are needed, perhaps from other therapists and agencies. Beyond this, our experience helps us to be proactive in anticipating problems and making arrangements to, wherever possible, prevent these problems from occurring.

5 Relationship: Working with colleagues and in teams

This performance area is about working effectively with other professionals to ensure patient care, including the sharing of information with colleagues.

In this part of the competence framework, we move beyond communication skills as applied to the consultation and into the area of communicating more widely with fellow professionals and members of the team. It is best not to see this as an entirely separate skill-set to that required for consultation, but as another application of it.

As for many other behaviours that we learn in order to become effective GPs, it helps to think about our attitudes. These often underpin our behaviour in the sense that if our *attitude* is appropriate, many behaviours often flow naturally. The converse is also true. This is not really surprising if we remember that our attitudes and our motivations are very closely related. If we have appropriate attitudes, our motivations, which we usually don't think about but which operate automatically beneath the surface, will drive our behaviour in a useful direction.

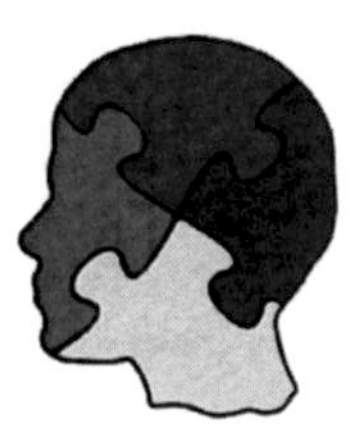

Joined up?
See p14

Just as teamworking skills are an extension of the communication skills developed in the consulting room, the mindset or attitude of teamworking is an extension of the 'partnership' mindset that we develop through our interactions with patients.

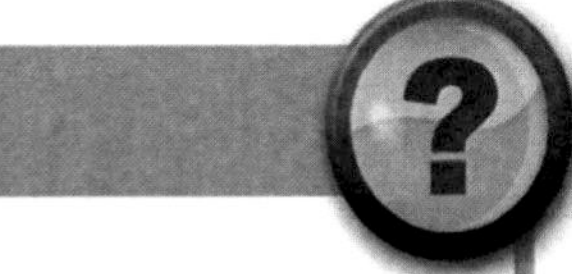

Using consulting skills in teamworking

Teamworking uses the skills acquired in consulting. Which of these do you feel are particularly important?

To answer this, think about the holistic dimension of patient care and how GPs involve the patient's family, friends, employer etc. in the teamwork that is often needed to deal with more significant problems.

The need for teamwork

It used to be the case that to achieve the targets that were required of it, a practice needed good decision-making, strong leadership and a well-organised infrastructure. Many 'teams' began life with this pyramidal hierarchy in which doctors and managers were at the top, nurses in the middle and the receptionists at the bottom.

As we will explore below, this system does not encourage individuals, and therefore organisations, to grow into modern teams that are capable of moving from dealing with demands in fire-fighting mode, to anticipating and planning for change. Such growth is vital, partly because of the increasing complexity and pace of change of primary care but also because ensuring others of the quality of our care (through clinical governance), can only be achieved through joint planning and sharing of responsibilities.

Let's take the experience of the first National Service Framework on coronary heart disease (CHD) to illustrate this point. To deliver primary and secondary prevention in line with the framework may require members of the practice to contribute in the following ways:

- **GPs:** reviewing the evidence, altering clinical management
- **Practice nurses**: revising CHD, Hypertension and diabetes protocols
- **Community pharmacist**: reviewing practice prescribing and the formulary
- **Practice manager**: planning, reviewing resources and logistics, coordinating needs- assessment
- **Receptionists**: providing information and feedback, directing and booking patients appropriately
- **Audit coordinator**: auditing diagnosis & management of hypertension, prescribing of aspirin & statins, recording of lifestyle factors etc.
- **Health visitors**: providing lifestyle advice, smoking cessation clinics
- **Community nurses**: providing baseline data, lifestyle advice, taking blood samples etc. Some will also have specialised functions such as heart failure management in the community.

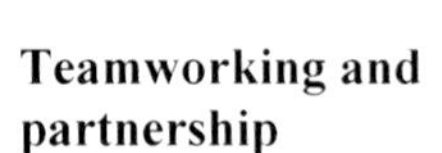

Teamworking and partnership

We need to move beyond thinking of team members as ancillary workers, called in to help at our request. Instead, we should think of them as partners with appropriate status and responsibility in helping to contribute to *and shape* the patient's management.

Although we may have overall responsibility, this does not mean that we should also have exclusive ownership.

Empowering the team through our personal attitude is strongly motivating for them and through this, for ourselves.

This list is not exhaustive, and does not include the involvement of public and patients who we could regard as members of the widest team. The traditional 'top down' hierarchy is inappropriate because many of the tasks outlined above are better planned and delivered by the named groups in a co-ordinated fashion, with individuals being accountable to their task groups and through these to the wider team.

There are people with many talents within any general practice team, and it makes sense to use their skills to help the practice to flourish and to reduce risks. This can be done by encouraging their ideas, utilising their ability to spot potential problems before harm is caused. Think in terms of many hands making light work rather than too many cooks spoiling the broth!

What is a team?

In basic terms, a team is a group of individuals who work together to achieve a common purpose. We are good at defining the structure of a team in terms of the roles, responsibility and lines of accountability of those within it, but are less adept at looking at the environment within which teams operate. The latter is important because if we understand the factors that help or hinder teamwork, we are better able to understand why things go wrong and how they might be corrected, or better still, anticipated.

How can we build a successful team?

Teams exist at various levels. We are already familiar with uni-disciplinary teams, many of which work well because they are composed of people who understand and respect each other, share common values and have common goals. Integrated nursing teams and successful GP partnerships are good examples of these.

Multi-disciplinary teams face not only the generic problems of working in groups, but also the difficulties of relating to people who have different responsibilities, attitudes and priorities. Beyond multidisciplinary practice teams, there are locality teams such as commissioning groups that involve other practices whose circumstances, priorities and ways of working together may differ from our own.

For any of these teams to work well, they need to be able to:

- Share information
- Discuss & decide
- Prepare for change

The prospect of team development may seem daunting, but it need not be if we remember that the building blocks of every team are the individuals within it. If we spend time trying to ensure that our colleagues feel valued and are encouraged to contribute, then there will be much less need to spend time trying to solve the problems of a dysfunctional group. As we often say, prevention is better than cure!

What, then, do individuals need in order to achieve this happy state, and how might we help them? To answer this question, the much-quoted work of the psychologist Abraham Maslow gives us some ideas. *(Maslow, Abraham (1970) motivation and personality. Harper & Row: New York)*

He suggested that individuals develop by meeting their needs in relation to a hierarchy. The sequential nature referred to the fact that meeting one need empowered the individual to develop at the next level. The word hierarchy was important, because Maslow suggested that no matter how developmentally advanced an individual might be, progress would be impaired if a lower-order need resurfaced. Hence, planning to become a GP trainer (a self-actualisation need) might be put on hold if we became ill (a biological need). This hierarchy of development can also be used to consider how groups of individuals, or teams, grow. Let us do this by considering the following table:

Maslow's hierarchy applied to team development		
Need	**Interpretation**	**How might we help?**
Self-actualisation needs (Top of the hierarchy)	Becoming self-confident and aware of our potential. Setting and meeting our own goals. Helping others to develop their potential	• Encouraging others to set goals • Empowering groups to consider new challenges • Providing a mechanism to monitor and applaud progress e.g. appraisal
Esteem needs	Being made to feel worthwhile by others Having our achievements recognised	• Encouraging groups to express ideas, train themselves and contribute to the practice • Rewarding effort through positive feedback and praise
Affiliation needs	Feeling wanted Being able to confide our thoughts	• Being willing to listen to group representatives • Ensuring confidentiality • Encouraging friendliness • Socialising
Safety needs	Feeling secure, free from anxiety Knowing the boundaries of our responsibility	• Making the remit of the group clear • Ensuring that individuals know their roles and responsibilities within the group • Providing resources, support and advocacy for the group
Biological needs (Bottom of the hierarchy)	Feeling physically comfortable	• Providing comfortable conditions in which to meet • Ensuring that people are not cold, hungry or tired

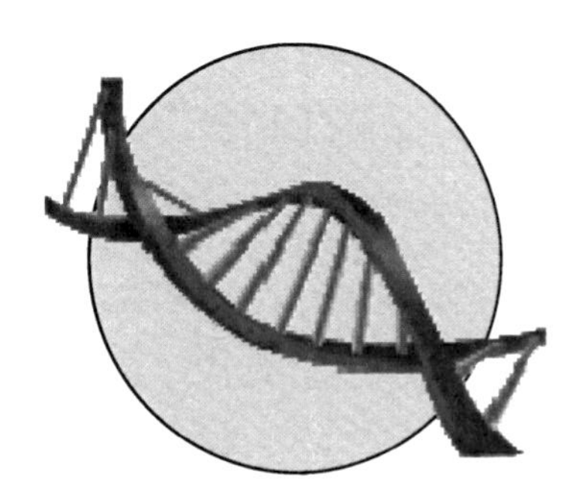

This framework presents the environment or culture within which successful teams grow. Many of the ideas that general practice uses are borrowed from Industry and in the commercial world, organisations known for their team building have no reservations about expressing a positive corporate culture. We might think of doing the same, not in the rather passé manner of the 'mission statement' where we promise to respect everyone and their budgie, but in practical ways such as those illustrated in the tables.

To remind ourselves of the deeper features that are being tested in this part of 'relationships', see page 24. Many of these competencies are to do with communication, but they also include the ability to take a lead role and to delegate appropriately.

We will now look at the specifics of teamworking through the MRCGP competence framework.

Needs Further Development	Competent for licensing	Excellent	
Meets contractual obligations to be available for patient care.	Provides appropriate availability to colleagues.	Anticipates situations that might interfere with availability and ensures that patient care is not compromised	**1**

This first progression illustrates how we move from:

Being around as required by our employment contract or partnership agreement, but not being more proactive in making ourselves more accessible to colleagues.

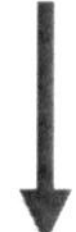

Being present, but also being *available* by letting colleagues know the best times to be contacted and by tailoring that availability according to the circumstances.

Looking ahead to periods when the usual availability may be disrupted, for example through planned absence from work or through changes to the usual rota such as at Christmas/New Year, and then making arrangements for teamwork to continue effectively, particularly for patients such as the terminally ill.

Needs Further Development	Competent for licensing	Excellent
Appropriately utilises the roles and abilities of other team members.	Works co-operatively with the other members of the team, seeking their views, acknowledging their contribution and using their skills appropriately.	Encourages the contribution of colleagues and contributes to the development of the team.

2

This second progression illustrates how we move from:

Understanding the roles and particular skills of team members and then using these skills appropriately.

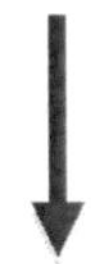

A much more active involvement with the team in which we discuss the management of cases and seek views and opinions before decisions are made. We also seek to improve relationships and teamworking by giving credit where credit is due.

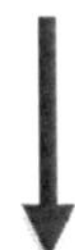

At the most developed stage, we show a deeper understanding of how to build and support a healthcare team. We play an active role in improving teamworking, particularly by encouraging colleagues to make use of existing opportunities and by creating new opportunities for team members to contribute.

Looking at each of the word pictures in turn:

Appropriately utilises the roles and abilities of other team members.

Even at this basic level, the curriculum encourages us to get to know other members of the team as *people* as well as practitioners. Obviously, it is important to know the roles of various team members so that we don't refer inappropriately. We also need to know where these roles overlap. For example, a patient with postnatal depression may be referred to the counsellor, but the health visitor may also need to know so that mother and child can be supported and PND can be looked for in future pregnancies.

For some problems, a whole range of therapists may be available to choose from. For example, eye problems could involve optometrists, ophthalmologists, orthoptists, school health services, community eye clinics and social workers. To take an example from rheumatology, problems may require the help of the rheumatology GPwSI, physiotherapist, podiatrist, osteopath, chiropractor, orthopaedic surgeon or rheumatologist. Knowing who does what and in what timescale, is no mean achievement and is important to get right partly for the patient's sake but also because inappropriate referrals waste scarce resources.

Developing our teamworking skills

How would you find out whether you were using the skills of team members appropriately?

Many significant events involve a breakdown in communication. Think of significant events that you have been involved in and ask yourself whether better communication between team members might have made any difference.

What do you think are your own teamworking weaknesses and how could you improve?

GPs have a vital role with chronic disease management and it is our job to ensure that the appropriate team is used and supported. To take diabetes as an example, the team would include diabetes nurse specialists, dieticians, district nurses, community matrons, chiropodists and opticians.

The word picture refers to the 'abilities' of team members in addition to their roles and this implies that we should be alert for how team members perform. To use team members appropriately and to assist their personal development, we should also find out what their particular areas of interest are. For example, the practice receptionists are the cornerstone of a well-functioning practice and as well as having a broad range of skills, may have particular areas of expertise such as knowing how to search the database for audit purposes.

Works co-operatively with the other members of the team, seeking their views, acknowledging their contribution and using their skills appropriately.

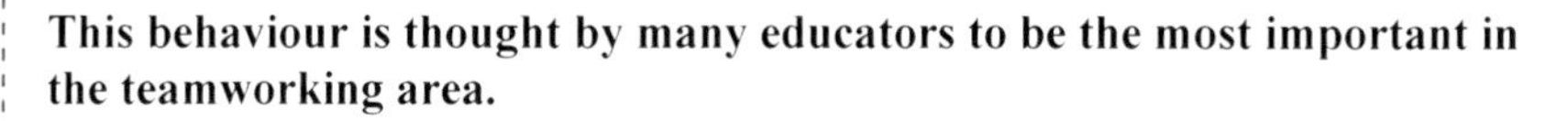

This behaviour is thought by many educators to be the most important in the teamworking area.

This competency is really about working in partnership with team members on patient management. At times, this may mean taking on the responsibilities of leading a team with a particular task. At others, it may mean responding to the requests of other team members, i.e. being delegated to.

In all situations, working co-operatively requires us to know how to communicate effectively, for example by knowing how best to contact particular members of the team by telephone, e-mail message book and so on.

Encourages the contribution of colleagues and contributes to the development of the team.

Really effective team members are not people who wait to take orders. They are proactive, taking steps to understand how well the team is working and how it can be made more effective. This requires us to understand the different roles that comprise an effective team and know how to build confidence and ability in team members through training and feedback. We also need to understand our own preferences regarding our role and develop certain specific skills that help with teamworking such as:

- Delegating tasks appropriately.
- Understanding how to motivate people.
- Conducting an appraisal interview.
- Organising an effective meeting.
- Chairing a meeting.
- Managing a project.

Needs Further Development	Competent for licensing	Excellent
When requested to do so, appropriately provides information to others involved in the care of the patient.	Communicates proactively with team members so that patient care is not compromised. In relation to the circumstances, chooses an appropriate mode of communication to share information with colleagues and uses it effectively.	Encourages the contribution of colleagues and contributes to the development of the team.

3

This third progression illustrates how we move from:

A basic level of responsiveness, providing information to other team members on request. Because we understand the roles, we can appropriately target information to different team members. Additionally, we avoid indiscriminately sharing sensitive information, where this is not needed by the team member.

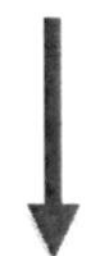

A more proactive approach, in which we keep team members updated without being asked to do so. We also understand how best to communicate with team members and how quickly to do so as guided by the circumstances. 'Effective communication' does not just apply to managing the problem, but also includes sharing information about the outcomes of patient management, including complaints and significant events, not forgetting *positive* feedback of course!

Looking at each of the word pictures in turn:

When requested to do so, appropriately provides information to others involved in the care of the patient.

This basic-level competency concerns our ability to respond appropriately to those team members in primary and secondary care who need to know about the patient's management. Increasingly these days, this can include a variety of community workers and agencies such as community matrons, hospital at home practitioners, emergency care practitioners and so on.

Part of our role is to ensure that information is shared appropriately and securely, which may mean taking extra steps to preserve confidentiality such as confirming that the request is coming from a legitimate source.

There are some basics about the information that is needed by the team. In an ideal world, team members:

- Are informed of those things that have a direct bearing on their work
- Do not receive information that they do not require (information overload and confidentiality risk)
- Are presented with information in an understandable form
- Do not get conflicting or inaccurate information
- Know where to get information when needed

To this list of 'rights' we could add one *responsibility*, which is for team members (i.e. all the team, not just ourselves) to pass on relevant information in an appropriate way to those who need to know.

Developing good communication in the team

It can be all too easy to blame other people for not communicating well, for example hospital wards and outpatient departments.

Once you have got over your irritation, what could you do to improve the situation?

Which of your suggestions have you personally implemented?

Communicates proactively with team members so that patient care is not compromised.

Being proactive means thinking ahead and anticipating situations in which patient care could be compromised. This applies to any situation in which patient care is dependent on good teamworking, for example chronic disease management and palliative care. Our responsibility as GPs is to make sure that continuity of care, communication between team members and clarity of responsibility is maintained.

To give a simple example from palliative care, we may need to let out-of-hours services know about the patient so that an inappropriate emergency visit or attempt at admitting the patient to hospital is avoided. Similarly, we may need to arrange for a colleague to take over medical responsibility whilst we are on holiday and to let the team know of this arrangement.

Although not explicitly mentioned, the patient and the patient's family/carers should be thought of as part of the team and kept informed to the appropriate degree. Good teamwork means that care is smooth, without unpleasant and unnecessary surprises. When this happens, patients and their families feel confident, which enhances trust and (importantly) promotes health by reducing avoidable distress.

Unfortunately, poor communication between team members is rife. This is partly because teams cross boundaries between hospital and community, have members who are answerable to different bosses and have cultures that don't always concord. As GPs, we are usually the people with the most experience and understanding of teamworking and although challenging, we are therefore often the best people to take responsibility for ensuring, for the reasons stated above, that it happens well.

In relation to the circumstances, chooses an appropriate mode of communication to share information with colleagues and uses it effectively.

In the simplest form, this may mean using the computer, telephone and fax machines appropriately and securely. Depending on the urgency of the situation, we may choose to ring for an appointment rather than send a letter. Similarly, services are geared up to respond to different levels of urgency. We need to be aware of this so that we can use (for example) emergency services, rapid-access clinics such as for chest pain or suspected stroke, and cancer diagnostic clinics appropriately.

In some situations, our skill depends upon recognising situations where particular protocols come into play and where temporary teams need to be convened. For example, dealing effectively with suspected child abuse involves: recognising the clinical features, knowing about local arrangements for child protection, referring effectively and playing a part in assessment and continuing management, including prevention of further abuse in the patient and family. There are many communication issues that are involved in this scenario, including how to raise the issue with the family whilst maintaining their trust and how to raise awareness in colleagues without encouraging prejudice.

'Sharing information' also refers to jointly discussing patient management as part of professional development and risk management. We may therefore contribute to regular significant event audits and case reviews. Additionally in some circumstances such as suspected adverse reactions to drugs and suspected infectious disease, we should consider reporting our experience more widely to regional or national units.

We have now completed the 'Relationship' cluster of the competence framework; as you can see, it wasn't too difficult to grasp. In the next section we will start thinking about 'Diagnostics' which brings together our core clinical skills.

Diagnostics

6 Diagnostics: Overview of the performance areas

'Diagnostics' is the second of the RDMp clusters and is made up of four domains from the competence framework, these being:

- Data gathering & interpretation
- Making a diagnosis/making decisions
- Clinical management
- Managing medical complexity

The process is not difficult to understand and briefly we can describe it in terms of a continuum of:

Being able to ask the right questions.......... from the right people (which will include colleagues) ... gather information from questions, investigations & examinations in order to:

decide which information is the most relevant and important..... generate ideas from ourselves and from others....... decide which of these ideas are the most important in order to:

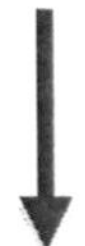

bring the strands together in a defensible plan

Because of our medical training, the focus of 'diagnostics' is on medical problems and clinical management. However, as GPs our problem-solving skills are applied much more widely. Therefore, the competencies that are discussed in most of this section can be transposed to non-clinical problems that crop up in any of the other areas of medical practice, for example relationship problems, management problems and issues concerning professionalism. These competencies can also be used to help us deal with problems that relate to ourselves as well as to others.

This cluster describes the heart of our clinical work as general practitioners.

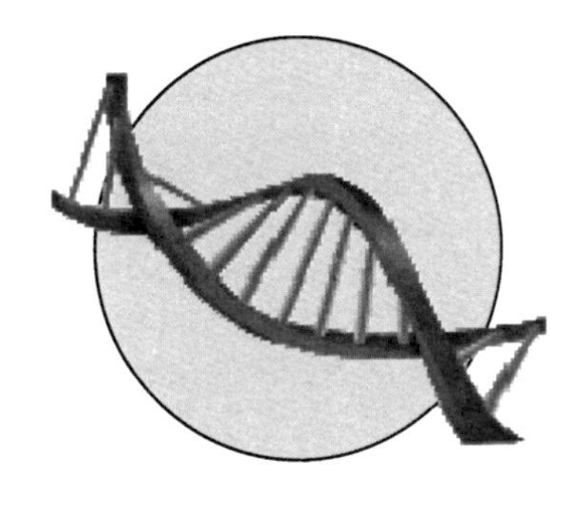

The deeper features are our DNA. Although few in number, they underpin all the behaviours described in the competence framework and are described in terms of knowledge, skills, attitudes and personal qualities. The behaviours being tested in the 'Diagnostics' section are shown in the table below, where the categories indicate the degree of weighting.

	Data gathering & interpretation	Making a diagnosis/ making decisions	Clinical management	Managing medical complexity
Clinical expertise	High	High	High	Medium
Problem-solving skills	Low	High	Low	Medium
Empathy & sensitivity			Low	Medium
Organisation & planning		Low	Low	Low

The behaviours are shown in the left-hand column. We will describe these in greater detail to clarify what they are. As you read them, use the table to cross-reference them to the domains that they underpin. This will increase your understanding and help you to develop the skills you need for each area of performance. The weighting will help you here. For example, 'managing medical complexity' requires empathy and sensitivity, whereas gathering data and making a diagnosis do not.

If you are (or your trainee is) having a problem with performance in a domain, look at the underlying deeper features for guidance on where the problem might lie and therefore which behaviours need working on.

Clinical expertise

- Understanding what information is needed to make a clinical decision and obtaining/eliciting this to the appropriate degree from patients and from colleagues.
- Not overlooking important information when this arises.
- Identifying the key issues and priorities, include the impact of the main problem on other patient problems and vice versa.
- Being able to understand the problem without having to see the full picture
- Knowing which are the appropriate options particularly in relation to possible diagnoses, tests and management approaches.
- Being able to generate a wide enough range of options, particularly with diagnoses and management approaches.
- Making judgements by collating information in a systematic manner and avoiding acting hastily.
- Looking ahead and anticipating the effect that problems might have on each other. Making plans to monitor for these and thereby minimize adverse consequences.

Problem-solving skills

- Showing the capacity to think analytically and work systematically
- Thinking flexibly around an issue, avoiding a narrow or dogmatic approach.
- Being able to see the wood from the trees and thereby identify the key issues
- Being able to suggest a workable outcome
- Being open to new ideas, possibilities and approaches

Empathy and sensitivity:

- Showing interest and understanding, when responding to the needs and concerns of patients and team members.
- Being open and non-judgemental.
- Taking active measures to include people in discussion and to work cooperatively with them.
- Using tone of voice and body language to indicate warmth and thereby encourage people to contribute.
- Taking steps to create a safe and trusting atmosphere through language, demeanour and behaviour.

Organisation & planning

- Being able to think ahead, plan and prepare, for example with management planning and clinical follow-up.
- Being able to build-in contingencies, for example clinical safety nets
- Being able to coordinate actions, monitor and set new priorities if the situation demands, for example when the unexpected happens.
- Being able to understand and work within the constraints, especially personal constraints and the limitations of the system and resources.

Making clinical decisions

In general terms, what types of information do you feel are needed in a GP encounter to make a clinical decision?
It is said that part of the GPs expertise is to *tolerate* uncertainty whereas hospital specialists aim to *reduce* uncertainty. In what ways do you agree and disagree with this statement?

When might you decide to tolerate uncertainty rather than reduce it?

Using probabilities

GPs need to relate their decision-making to the prevalence & incidence of disease in the community.

What information would you require about the community and about the practice in order to be able to do this?

7 Diagnostics: Data-gathering and interpretation

This performance area is about the gathering and use of data for clinical judgement, the choice of examination and investigations and their interpretation.

Needs Further Development	Competent for licensing	Excellent	
Obtains information from the patient that is relevant to their problem.	Systematically gathers information, using questions appropriately targeted to the problem. Makes appropriate use of existing information about the problem and the patient's context.	Proficiently identifies the nature and scope of enquiry needed to investigate the problem.	1

This first progression is principally about the history and illustrates how we move from:

Simply gathering information from the patient without seeking out what is already known or using a systematic and efficient approach to gather information.

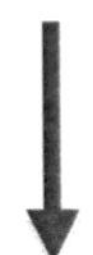

Showing the ability to use a targeted rather than blunderbuss approach, deciding what reliance can be placed on information that is already available and focusing any further enquiries on the problem.

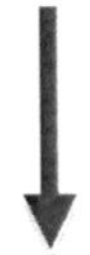

Having identified the problem, being able to quickly and fluently decide how far-ranging and probing the further enquiries need to be to adequately investigate the problem.

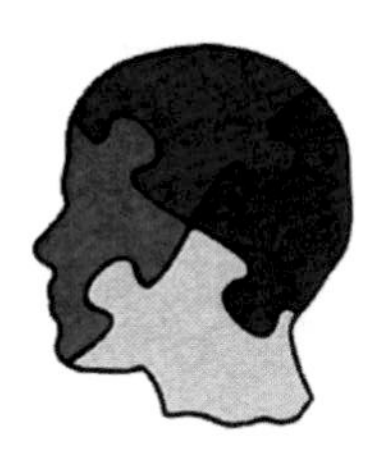

Joined up?
See p14

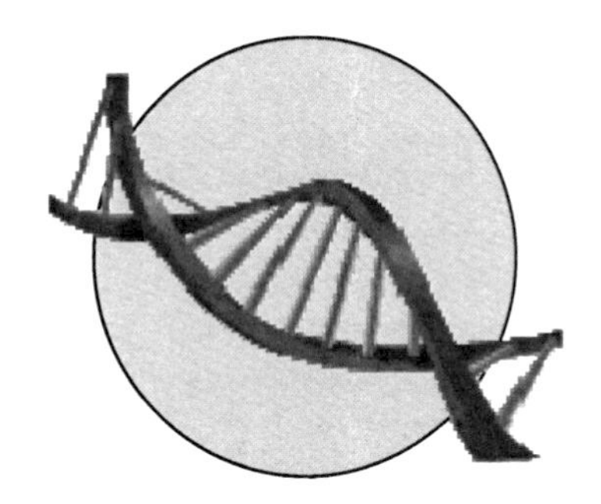

Which aspects of our DNA, our deeper features, are particularly important in Data gathering & interpretation ? If we look back at the competencies for the 'Diagnostics' section (page 60), we see that clinical expertise is heavily represented, followed by problem-solving skills. It is important to remember that 'data' is much wider than numbers and technical information and includes thoughts, opinions and judgements. In addition, data-gathering is the fuel for the problem-solving machine. It is therefore needed not just at the outset (for example, when the patient initially presents), but throughout the problem-solving process.

Looking at each of the word pictures from the first progression in turn:

Obtains information from the patient that is relevant to their problem.

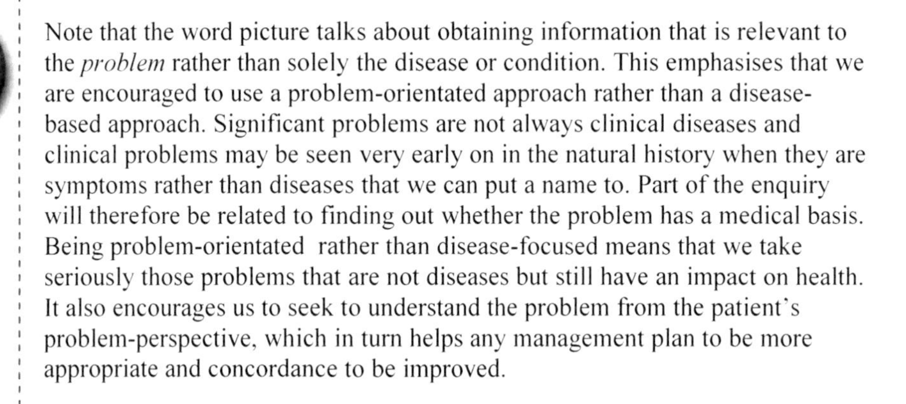

Note that the word picture talks about obtaining information that is relevant to the *problem* rather than solely the disease or condition. This emphasises that we are encouraged to use a problem-orientated approach rather than a disease-based approach. Significant problems are not always clinical diseases and clinical problems may be seen very early on in the natural history when they are symptoms rather than diseases that we can put a name to. Part of the enquiry will therefore be related to finding out whether the problem has a medical basis. Being problem-orientated rather than disease-focused means that we take seriously those problems that are not diseases but still have an impact on health. It also encourages us to seek to understand the problem from the patient's problem-perspective, which in turn helps any management plan to be more appropriate and concordance to be improved.

Systematically gathers information, using questions appropriately targeted to the problem.

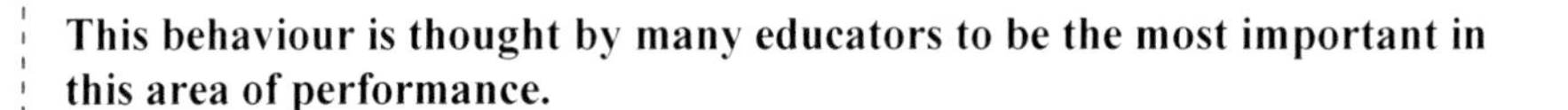

This behaviour is thought by many educators to be the most important in this area of performance.

Being systematic is very important and is looked for closely, particularly in CSA. Examiners need to feel that the candidate can be trusted to adopt a rational approach when faced with a problem. This is more important than just 'being right' in the sense that if the candidate suggests an appropriate diagnosis or management option, this must have its roots in rational enquiry and must not just appear from nowhere like a rabbit pulled from a hat.

Examples of systematic approaches are:

- The logical questioning used to investigate abdominal pain, allowing a doctor to make a diagnosis of irritable bowel syndrome by positively excluding other more serious conditions.
- The use of rating scales and questionnaires to establish the diagnosis of depression and rate its severity.
- The construction of a family tree by taking and interpreting a family history based on the knowledge of simple inheritance patterns.

'Targeting questions' often takes place in a different phase of the consultation, when communication moves from being inclusive and open to becoming more doctor-centred and closed. It is often better to signpost this phase to patients so that they do not feel distanced or, in a negative sense, interrogated.

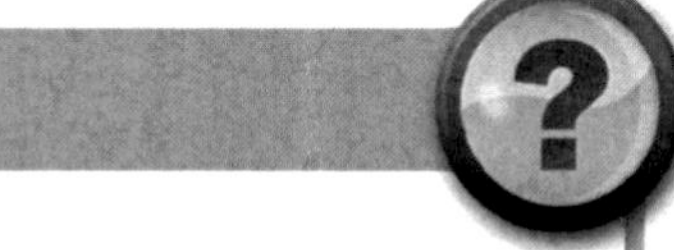

Whose problem is it?

When the problem has been identified and accepted by the patient, then further questions are likely to be accepted and responded to. Compare this to the frequent situation in which doctors pursue their own clinical agenda without adequately involving the patient.

Without explanation, preferably early on in the consultation, patients may not understand the purpose of questioning and can be reticent, obstructive or even angry. They may feel that we have not heard them or are ignoring their concerns.

For example, a patient may complain of pain in the left arm. Without explanation, enquiries about smoking, diabetes and exercise may seem puzzling or even pointless to the patient, whereas they would not to another doctor.

Makes appropriate use of existing information about the problem and the patient's context.

Making use of existing information means that once we have initial ideas about the problem, we look to see what information is available that might shed further light. This includes assessing to what degree this information can be relied upon and therefore whether previous history, examination and investigations need to be repeated or added to.

How would you make use of information about the patient's context?

Context is a broad term. At one level, it may refer to the patient's occupational, social and cultural background. Knowledge of the patient's occupation may modify the differential diagnosis and will almost certainly influence the management plan. For instance, back pain in a non-manual worker may not be a threat to livelihood in the way that it could be for a labourer. Occupational exposure may make some lung diseases more likely and a 'faint' will have different implications for an HGV driver than a bank clerk.

'Gender' is another example of context. The curriculum teaches us to recognise that men consult less frequently, have more illness and are generally more reluctant to admit a problem exists. Male sex should therefore lower our threshold for suspicion of significant disease (also see page 72 for a more general discussion of probability)

Proficiently identifies the nature and scope of enquiry needed to investigate the problem.

We must decide the range and depth of enquiry that is required. This means:

- Formulating a differential diagnosis,
- Identifying which differentials are more significant (perhaps in terms of risk) than others
- Deciding which questions are needed to explore these possibilities
- Deciding the range and depth of questions needed to exclude unlikely but serious alternatives
- Prioritising the questions appropriately, on the basis of the above

This behaviour falls in the 'excellent' bracket because we have to undertake this sequence proficiently, i.e. quickly and fluently, which requires considerable expertise when the differential diagnosis is extensive or complex.

For example, we may be presented with difficult symptoms such as dizziness or headache, where there are multiple differentials, some of which are serious. Efficient problem-solving will depend upon having a structured and logical approach to questioning and diagnosis.

Once again, the exploration must occur with the consent and co-operation of the patient, which means that we must explain what we are asking, be alert to cues and explain our findings.

Assessor's corner: systematic questioning

Systematic questioning is easy to spot when the style is more of an interrogation. More fluent doctors tend not ask all the relevant questions in one go, but bring them in at appropriate points, building up a picture throughout the consultation.

Look out for red flag symptoms and signs. These should not be missed and should normally trigger targeted questioning.

Assessor's corner: using available information

There are many sources of information with the main ones being from the patient and medical records.

Does the trainee make use of this information and try to link it with the patient's problem, thereby putting the problem in context?

Needs Further Development	Competent for licensing	Excellent
Employs examinations and investigations that are broadly in line with the patient's problem. Identifies abnormal findings and results.	Chooses examinations and targets investigations appropriately. Identifies the implications of findings and results.	Uses an incremental approach, basing further enquiries, examinations and tests on what is already known and what is later discovered.

2

What types of test might we be expected to know about?

Targeting investigations means understanding the indications for a test and also knowing which tests are best, based on availability, predictive value and patient acceptability. **Examples include:**

Blood tests

The indications for plain x-rays, ultrasound, CT and MRI

Knowledge of secondary care investigations and treatment, e.g. endoscopy, abdominal imaging, biopsy, ERCP in abdominal investigations, EEG and nerve conduction studies in neurological problems, slit lamp investigations and IOP measurement in ophthalmological problems.

This second progression leads on from history taking and is concerned with physical examination and investigations. The progression illustrates how we move from:

Targeting examinations and investigations to the patient's problem; recognising when tests are abnormal, even if we do not fully understand the implications.

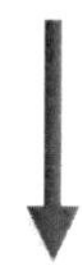

Deciding what reliance can be placed on available data and focusing any further questions, examination and tests on the problem. Additionally, understanding what the implications of abnormal results might be.

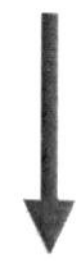

Taking a stepwise approach, monitoring the situation and tailoring further tests to our evolving understanding of the problem.

Looking at each of the word pictures in turn:

Employs examinations and investigations that are broadly in line with the patient's problem.

There is an assumption here that examinations and investigations are necessary. This is not always the case and there are situations in which investigation may delay the appropriate action. Obviously, emergency admission is one such. Another is when the situation is not an emergency but could deteriorate during the investigation period. For example, the curriculum warns us that investigation may delay referral in suspected head and neck cancer.

Identifies abnormal findings and results.

At the 'needs further development' level, we need to recognize when the data suggests abnormality. For many tests, this may not be a challenge as laboratories increasingly highlight abnormal results, showing the normal range and even suggesting possible causes or recommended action. However, there are many other pieces of information that can't be highlighted in this way and require baseline knowledge on our part.

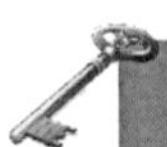

Chooses examinations and targets investigations appropriately.

This behaviour is thought by educators to be particularly important

'Choosing examinations' means deciding which examinations are required to provide the information needed to include or exclude a diagnosis from the list of possibilities. Examining a patient in primary care is not the same as in hospital. There is not the same expectation that a full medical clerking will be undertaken with a top to toe examination. Also, time available is very short especially when we include the time taken for the patient to dress/undress. Making an appropriate choice is also influenced by patient consent and the need to maintain the patient's dignity.

In CSA, certain cases may require doctors to suggest or to undertake physical examination. Examiners will be looking for the ability to weigh the risks, think of the likelihood of examination contributing significantly to the diagnostic process and then choose appropriately, treating the patient with compassion and respect.

'Targeting investigations' requires us to decide upon appropriate tests for any particular problem. 'Investigations' can include questionnaires, such as dementia screens or depression inventories. When targeting investigations, we also need to take into account the cost-efficiency and cost-benefit of tests. Tests may sometimes be counter-productive if they distract us, e.g. by producing red-herrings. This can lead to patient harm as well as being a poor use of resources, so choosing tests carefully is important.

Identifies the implications of findings and results.

Clearly, we would be expected to understand the implications of a normal finding or test. With abnormal findings and tests, there will be implications for case management which may include: no further action, repeating the test, obtaining more information perhaps through further investigation and finally, referral. Another factor is the urgency with which any of the above need to be conducted.

In the workplace, we may repeat tests if they date from some time back, but may be quite happy with recent results. In CSA, there may be a temptation to repeat tests 'for safety's sake'. However, examiners are looking for the ability to 'make appropriate use of existing information' which means that it may be quite in order to accept results without repeating them. This also allows us to demonstrate our efficient use of resources.

Broadly speaking, abnormal findings and tests will modify our previous estimation of the probability of 'nothing being wrong' versus 'something being wrong', or one condition being more likely than another.

What other sorts of abnormality might we be asked to identify?

These might include abnormal physiological measurements such as temperature and blood pressure. You may also be expected to know how these numbers compare with guideline recommendations. For example, a BP that is normal for a non-diabetic individual may be too high in a diabetic.

Near patient tests such as urinalysis, blood glucose and ECG

Recognizing abnormalities includes identifying deviations from an acceptable trend. For example, deviations from growth centiles, simple spirometry results and trends in a serial peak flow chart.

'Abnormality' may also be recognized from a cluster of measurements. For instance, coronary heart disease risk is derived from a multifactorial assessment of physiological and lifestyle factors in an individual.

Data may also be used to assess health care, e.g. a comparison of standardised mortality rates between the practice population and neighbouring populations.

'Probability' is not simply an intellectual notion. The most significant way in which we can demonstrate our understanding of the implications of findings and results is in the way we *explain* these to the patient. This includes communicating the probabilities and then checking that they have been correctly understood.

Uses an incremental approach, basing further enquiries, examinations and tests on what is already known and what is later discovered.

The key skill here is to use a stepwise approach, which implies having a mental map of how the problem might evolve. It also implies constantly monitoring the patient's progress to look for deviations from the expected path. When deviations occur, further information may be needed (such as examinations and investigations) and the map may need to be modified. We therefore can't afford to have a rigid approach or a dogmatic mindset. Instead, we need to have our antennae perpetually twitching for feedback and further information and to have a flexible and forgiving approach.

Why forgiving? Because rather than feel upset that the initial diagnosis or management plan is shown to be wrong, we should *expect* not to be immediately correct and should expect to modify our ideas and plans as the problem unfolds. This approach means that we don't threaten our self-esteem through inappropriate expectations and that we remain vigilant, rarely drawing a line under a problem. This is good for us and good for patient safety.

Given that we have to work in much more uncertain conditions than hospital doctors, this mindset is appropriate. Incidentally, it is usually well-understood by patients, who are more forgiving if doctors are open with them about the uncertainties and probabilities and if they are forewarned that ideas are likely to change as the journey progresses.

There are many examples of patient journeys in which time is used as a diagnostic tool (see page 72). Chronic neurological conditions like multiple sclerosis and Parkinson's disease are good examples of where this approach is essential. With any prolonged incremental journey, the importance of good communication, trust and partnership cannot be underestimated and is also an important part of risk management.

In what way could DNA rates be thought of as abnormal findings?

The point of this question is to illustrate that 'findings' can come from many sources. Practices notice when patients DNA appointments that they had booked and GPs may use this information to modify patient behaviour (or at least, to try!).

Sometimes the implications of this abnormal finding may be more significant. For example, if children fail to attend appointments this may trigger concern, given that they are reliant on parents and carers to make the appointment. Is the children's care an issue?

Could DNAs reflect a problem with the convenience of appointment times?

Tolerating uncertainty

The process of 'tolerating' does not simply mean stoically or lazily accepting a situation, but anticipating that some situations will be associated with a great deal of uncertainty and that steps can be taken to minimise this.

Using a stepwise approach to deal with chronic problems is a good example of a situation where uncertainty is inevitable and where good communication, partnership and follow-up can minimise the adverse effects

In the next chapter, we will see how the data that is gathered is then used for probably the most important skill that GPs have, which is to make justifiable decisions in situations of complexity and uncertainty.

8 Diagnostics: Making a diagnosis/ making decisions

This performance area is about a conscious, structured approach to decision-making.

This performance area follows on from data-gathering which is not an end in itself, but provides information for making diagnoses and making decisions. We can see that this area is not simply about the clinical arena, although this is the most important one. It also encompasses problem-solving more widely, where decisions have to be reached about problems that may not be clinical, but have an impact on health. For example, GPs often have to make decisions that are related to employment, housing and social benefits.

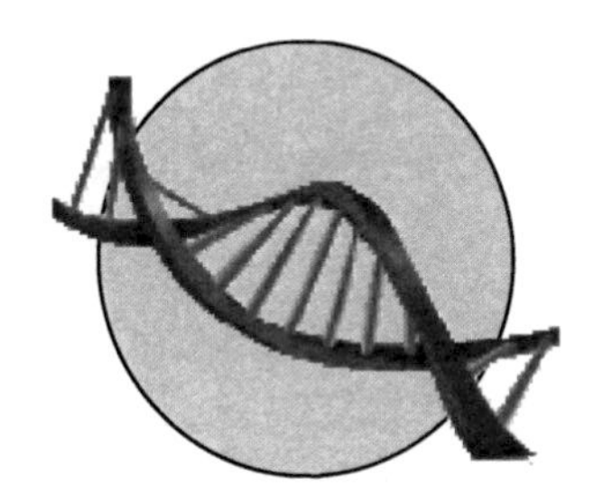

Which aspects of our DNA, our deeper features, are particularly important in making diagnoses and decisions? If we look back at the competencies for the 'Diagnostics' section (page 60), we see that clinical expertise and problem solving are equally important. In addition to these predictable elements, we gain a further insight by seeing that organisation and planning skills are also needed.

Needs Further Development	Competent for licensing	Excellent	
Taking relevant data into account, clarifies the problem and the nature of the decision required.	Addresses problems that present early and in an undifferentiated way by integrating information to aid pattern recognition. Uses time as a diagnostic tool. Uses an understanding of probability based on prevalence, incidence and natural history of illness to aid decision-making.	Uses methods such as models and scripts to identify patterns quickly and reliably. Uses an analytical approach to novel situations where probability cannot be readily applied.	**1**

This first progression is principally about building up a picture so that the nature and shape of a problem can be recognized or a clinical diagnosis made. We move from:

Using available information (from data gathering), finding out what the problem is and what is expected from us.

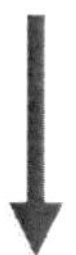

Collating information until a pattern emerges, using an understanding of probability. Allowing this process to take place over time so that the picture can be progressively better informed.

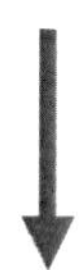

Using theoretical models and scripts built up through experience, to reliably anticipate what the pattern might be. Additionally, analysing the situation from first principles where shortcuts, based on knowledge of probability, are not available.

Using audit to make decisions

Taken more broadly, this word picture could be applied to decisions that are related to systems rather than people.

'Using relevant information to find out whether a problem exists' could be taken as a definition of audit. Doctors often use information relating to personal and practice performance to find out whether performance is significantly outside the acceptable range, which may mean that a problem exists.

In this situation, our 'decision' would be to work on individual performance, and/or on the performance of a system.

Looking at each of the word pictures in turn:

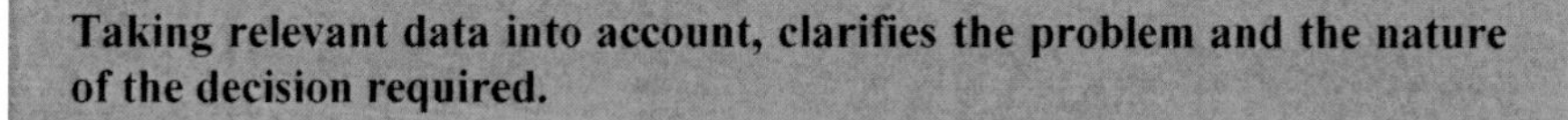

Taking relevant data into account, clarifies the problem and the nature of the decision required.

In a sense, the whole of this competency progression is about 'clarifying the problem'. At this basic level, what is required is that we make use of the available data and in broad terms, establish whether there is a problem that we can help with and if so, what sort of solution is possible. The 'solution' normally specifies the management plan and the degree of urgency.

For example, if we are unable to deal with the problem ourselves, the patient may need to be redirected or referred, perhaps urgently. Urgency can range from redirecting a patient with ear wax to a nurse for ear syringing/ referring a patient requesting a vasectomy to a specialist clinic/ calling an ambulance for crushing chest pain. In these examples, the decision that we make is straightforward and does not require significant negotiation with the patient.

Much more often, the patient has a problem for which the cause is not yet known and therefore the management is unclear. In these situations, the decisions relate to determining the appropriate management options that can then be discussed with the patient.

Occasionally, what is required from us is not yet clear. This may be because someone has reported a problem on behalf of the patient, but the patient has not yet been seen.

Alternatively, the patient has a problem but doesn't yet know whether our help is needed. For example,' lethargy' is a common symptom that may reflect the patient's circumstances rather than be an indicator of disease. Because patients have continuing relationships with their doctors, it is not uncommon for them to attend early on simply to discuss their symptoms before it becomes clear whether or not a medical problem exists. The 'decision' in this situation might simply be to wait and see.

Sometimes, no medical problem exists and the patient simply requires reassurance. The curriculum points out that part of our role is to identify symptoms that are within the normal range and require no treatment e.g. cyclical blocking of the nose, senile rhinorrhoea and small neck lymph nodes in children who are well.

Occasionally a problem *does* exist, but not in the way that the patient imagines. For example, patients may somatise, believing that symptoms such as musculoskeletal pain or weakness are due to physical illness, when in fact they may be due to psychological causes. Here, our decision is not so much how to treat physical symptoms as how to manage the somatisation.

'Taking relevant data into account' includes being aware of the patient's context. Because solutions are specific to particular contexts, this information is vital if the appropriate way forward is to be found. (see page 64)

As we can see, as well as taking facts and figures into account, this competency is strongly influenced by consulting skills and particularly by our ability to question, listen and keep alert for cues. Sometimes, the most significant problem only manifests itself as a hidden agenda and is therefore only disclosed to doctors who have curiosity and show the patient that they are interested in finding out more.

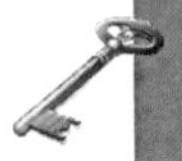

Addresses problems that present early and in an undifferentiated way by integrating information to aid pattern recognition.

This is a key competency. In general practice, many problems present in an undifferentiated state, i.e. well before it becomes clear what the information represents. This skill involves being aware of patterns such as the natural histories of common diseases and then purposefully bringing information together to see if it fits a particular pattern.

The skill also involves being able to see what *is* there, rather than what we would like to see. It's all too easy in clinical practice to shoehorn the clues into a preferred pattern, but this runs the risk of treating the patient on the basis of a wrong diagnosis. Worse still, there is the risk of *not* treating a more serious diagnosis which may be emerging, but has been overlooked. To give an example, a child with poor weight gain diagnosed as a nutritional problem, may in fact be the victim of child abuse.

Alcoholism is a good example of a condition that presents an undifferentiated way.

Question: how can alcoholism be spotted earlier from the records?

The manifestation of alcohol problems include:

- **physical:** accidents, victim of violence, obesity, dyspepsia, erectile dysfunction, fits, foetal alcohol syndrome, liver damage, anaemia, neurological and central nervous system problems
- **psychological:** anxiety, depression, attempted suicide
- **social:** loss of employment, disorderly conduct, domestic violence, drink–driving, relationship problems or breakdown

Tip: aiding pattern recognition

Integrating information is much easier than hitherto thanks to computers and this can help us to recognise patterns much earlier. The process is dependent upon coding significant pieces of information such as attendances, problems, symptoms, tests and investigations.

Try looking back in the notes, prompted by a significant diagnosis such as bowel cancer and ask yourself 'Could this have been diagnosed earlier based on the information in the records?' If so, how could the data have been collated or coded better to make earlier diagnosis more likely?

Get in the habit of looking at previous consultations that have been coded with the same presenting symptom. This often makes the pattern clearer, prevents unnecessary tests and reduces inappropriate delays in treatment.

Another example of integrating information is to search records of family members to look for commonalities that might suggest genetic or environmental factors.

Tip: Improving our diagnostic use of time

Using time appropriately is dependent upon both competence and confidence. We can't rely upon confidence (unfortunately, poor doctors are often overconfident), but we can all work on our competence no matter how experienced or inexperienced we are.

Ask your colleagues to let you know of patients, previously under your care with similar symptoms, in whom they make a diagnosis. Ask your colleagues to let you know of situations that turn urgent or acute where you had been managing the patient by 'watchful waiting'.

Where a condition has been diagnosed in which you are not confident about the natural history, look back to see how the condition evolved. Look at the information/tests that eventually proved useful in making the diagnosis and the stage in the natural history when the diagnosis became evident.

Try auditing those referrals that you make for an opinion, where the condition is not clear to you. Could there have been any advantage in using time for a little longer? If the referral is premature, what costs are incurred to the patient (financial, morbidity etc.) through unnecessary tests?

Uses time as a diagnostic tool.

Because so many significant problems evolve over time, it is both appropriate and unavoidable to use time to see the picture emerge. This doesn't mean that the time period is necessarily long. For example, we may use time to see whether abdominal pain is in fact appendicitis rather than gastroenteritis.

Using time safely depends on having a sound grasp of the important differential diagnoses, the probabilities of serious disease and knowledge of what red flags to look for. Red flags are particularly important because these help us to safely shortcut the decision-making process.

Sometimes, the symptoms fade away and no diagnosis is made. However, this information need not be lost if it is coded and as we have discussed, it may allow a future episode of similar symptoms to be connected to it, thus allowing a pattern to emerge (if one exists).

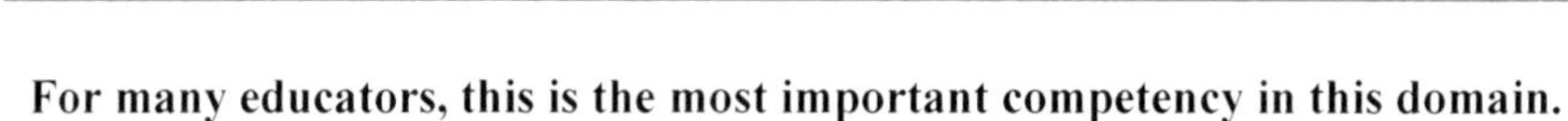

Uses an understanding of probability based on prevalence, incidence and natural history of illness to aid decision-making.

For many educators, this is the most important competency in this domain.

We can understand why, because without this skill we are not only unable to develop appropriate management plans for common conditions, but crucially, we are unable to 'diagnose normality' and therefore prevent unnecessary and potentially harmful treatment and the wastage of scarce resources.

The prevalence and incidence of disease is markedly different between primary and secondary care. Understanding the natural history is critical to developing appropriate management plans and even more importantly, to pick up on unexpected deviations from the anticipated evolution of a patient's problem. We often hear that 'common things occur commonly', but just as importantly, although rare things are rare, they still happen and they usually surface in primary care rather than in casualty.

Having said that, we should be wary of too often making fancy, esoteric diagnoses in the community. These may be appropriate in hospital, but this behaviour may reflect a lack of understanding of prevalence and probability in the 'unfiltered' population of primary care. We need to remember that when prevalence rates are low (as they are in the community) positive test results have a low predictive value. The opposite is true in hospital.

To understand probability, we need to understand our communities and the range and frequency of diseases that occur locally. With many conditions, the prevalence may not be much different to what is reflected in textbooks. However, the practice population may be skewed in a way that makes a significant difference. The practice age-sex profile might be unusual, for example with comparatively young populations in new conurbations and comparatively old populations in seaside retirement towns. Additionally, ethnic mix may change the incidence of chronic conditions like diabetes and heart disease and occupational hazards through local industry may raise the risk of, for instance, lung disease.

Probability also ties in with natural history and clinical associations in the sense that some conditions are unusual in the presence or absence of other factors. For example, new-onset migraine is unusual in an older adult and should make us think about more serious causes of headache. Likewise, Polymyalgia is uncommon with a normal ESR and might make us think of joint problems.

Sometimes probability has to be ignored in order to exclude important diagnoses. For example, several causes of headache are rare but important such as raised intracranial pressure, thunderclap headache (which may stem from subarachnoid haemmorhage, enlarging aneurysm or migraine) temporal arteritis, trigeminal neuralgia, herpes zoster and some cancers.

Sharing knowledge of probability with the patient, discussing what we think might happen and over what timescale, is a vital part of good safety netting.

Tip: spotting a problem with our performance

However good our interpersonal skills, patients get dissatisfied if we fail to clarify the problem by giving it a label.

Look out for dissatisfied patients and patients that you have seen who then seek a second opinion within the practice.

Also look at your late or missed diagnoses; could you have recognised a pattern sooner?

Uses methods such as models and scripts to identify patterns quickly and reliably.

This is a higher level of performance because mental models and illness scripts can only be developed through experience of making decisions in various contexts and through learning the patterns of presentation and evolution. Progressively superimposing new insights on a body of experience allows patterns to be recognised more quickly and reliably than occurs with a novice GP.

The downside of experience is that it tempts us to take unwarranted shortcuts, making assumptions and misinterpreting information consciously or unconsciously because it fits with a preconceived notion. This is why the word 'reliably' is important in this word picture.

Uses an analytical approach to novel situations where probability cannot be readily applied.

Sometimes, situations are new to us or even to medical practice, which means that no information on probability is available to guide our estimation of likelihood. Similarly, novel situations do not have an illness script to work from, so it is hard to manage the problem and to guide the patient. Nevertheless, as this word picture indicates, it is possible to use other approaches such as analyzing information to rule out other conditions. Additionally, we can look for associations, for example between symptoms and clinical findings, to see what conditions this might suggest.

To give a clinical example, a patient may present with flitting joint pains that don't fit any known pattern. There may be no joint swelling, but an analytical approach might reveal that the ESR,CRP and white cell count are raised, suggesting an inflammatory aetiology.

Needs Further Development	Competent for licensing	Excellent
Generates and tests an appropriate hypothesis. Makes decisions by applying rules or plans.	Revises hypotheses in the light of additional information. Thinks flexibly around problems, generating functional solutions.	No longer relies on rules alone but is able to use and justify discretionary judgement in situations of uncertainty.

2

The first progression within this domain concerned itself with pattern recognition. The second is concerned with the very important area of how we move from making decisions by applying rules to making decisions that are more reliant on our independent judgement. In today's rule-bound and accountable world, being able to do the latter is necessary, because many decisions in primary care are not amenable to algorithms, and don't have rules or guidelines that we can use to clarify or defend our decision. We could say that *the expertise of the GP begins where the algorithms end.*

Tip: learning how to critique the guidelines

Once you know the theory (page 156), pick out a couple of guidelines both national and local and see how they measure up. Talk to your colleagues about guidelines that they find helpful and ones that they don't. What are the reasons for the differences?

Have you come across any guidelines that you feel are questionable? What should you do about it?

In this second progression, we move from:

Coming up with reasonable suggestions as to what the problem/diagnosis might be and then using simple measures such as rules and guidelines to decide what should then be done.

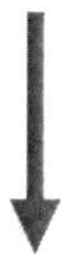

Becoming less rigid about sticking with initial plans and instead, being prepared to think again as the situation evolves.

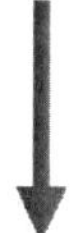

Recognising situations in which guidelines and rules don't exist or don't fully address the problem, and then using professional judgement to come up with justifiable approaches that are tailored to the situation.

Looking at each of the word pictures in turn:

Generates and tests an appropriate hypothesis.

In clinical terms, this often means generating an appropriate differential diagnosis. Put another way, the descriptor suggests that what we should *not* do is to jump to conclusions by making immediate assumptions.

Each of the differential diagnoses will have features that can be used to test out the likelihood of the condition being present. Our task is then to decide which differential diagnosis and test strategy to prioritise. The choice will be governed by a number of factors such as the availability of tests, their acceptability, affordability and so on. However, the most significant factor will be patient safety. Therefore, if a red flag indicator is present, this may well determine the priority for further tests.

For example, if the patient has a history for some months of being tight-chested and wheezy on exertion, but with chest pain radiating to the jaw at the same time, we might choose to use a trial of GTN spray rather than a bronchodilator to test out the hypothesis of angina rather than exercise-induced asthma. For clinical problems, we often call the 'hypothesis', the 'working diagnosis'.

Makes decisions by applying rules or plans.

Decision-making is probably the most important professional skill and this word picture is at one end of that continuum. At the other extreme lies our ability to use our own judgement when guidelines and protocols are not available. We might argue that rules and plans could include any systematic method that we use to reach a decision, including the 'clinical method' of history taking, examination and investigation. To some extent this is true, because at the very least we must demonstrate that have a systematic and rational approach to decision-making. However, this competency is principally about our ability to appropriately follow guidelines and protocols.

Part of the skill is in knowing *which* clinical conditions and problems are linked to rules and plans. This will vary not only with the condition, but with our geographical location. Therefore, we might expect to know and follow national service frameworks, but the impact of NICE guidelines and SIGN guidelines for example, will vary with the country we are working in. In addition, there will be local rules that we might be expected to follow such as referral policies, clinical care pathways, practice protocols and formularies.

Of course, it is not always possible to apply rules. Sometimes, there may be no guidelines available and of course, if a guideline exists but we are not aware of it, we would not be in a position to use it.

Revises hypotheses in the light of additional information.

The key abilities here are the willingness to keep an open mind and not assume that the first hypothesis was necessarily right. Don't make the facts fit the assumptions. For example, an itchy rash on the forearms might initially be treated as eczema and found to be unresponsive to topical steroids. If our mind is closed, we may fail to look closely for burrows and instead of treating for scabies, may instead increase the strength of the steroid preparation.

Question: when should probability be ignored?

Probability does not take account of the significance of any particular condition. Therefore, although rare things happen rarely, some of these rare diagnoses may be particularly serious. Red flags are a classic example of situations where probability is ignored in the interests of patient safety (and related to this, medicolegal risk).

Many doctors come across situations where no red flag is present, but where an internal alarm bell rings. This may relate to some previous experience that turned out to be serious, or to recognising something unusual about the current situation.

Because pattern recognition is a complex affair, these ' alarm bells' should not be ignored and in fairness, secondary care readily accept referrals on the basis of a hunch because they recognize that not infrequently, these hunches prove to be correct.

These clinical suspicions are worthy of being recorded in some way that does not worry the patient, but is clear to another clinician.

Learn to recognize and record your hunches and go back to the patient's records after a few months. Were you right, did something evolve and if so what have you learned?

Assessor's corner: does the doctor fail to revise the working diagnosis appropriately?

It may appear from discussion or from the records that only *one* diagnosis is being considered. A range of other options & differential diagnoses may not be forthcoming, suggesting a narrow mindset.

As new information becomes available that appears relevant to the problem, the trainee may not use this as a prompt to think again.

New information that seems *inconsistent or incompatible* with the working diagnosis may also be overlooked. In a worst-case scenario, red flag symptoms suggestive of an alternative (and serious) diagnosis may be ignored.

The worst consequences of this type of behaviour would be near misses, significant events, patient harm and patient complaints.

We may feel reluctant to commit ourselves to 'showing our thinking' in the medical records for a number of reasons. Sometimes, as in the scabies example above, this can be because we do not wish to alarm the patient. However, because conditions are often managed in modern primary care by more than one clinician, it can be helpful to see what *previous* clinicians considered in addition to their working diagnosis. This can act as a useful prompt to investigate further, treat differently or refer, and may prevent patients from being treated inappropriately for any longer than is unavoidable. In this sense, 'revising hypotheses' is a *team-based* activity and is facilitated by making the thinking processes of those involved in patient care, more explicit.

Thinks flexibly around problems, generating functional solutions.

This is thought by educators to be a particularly important competency.

Once the problem has been clarified, we move to the stage of creating management options. These options are not simply a list developed by ourselves and presented to the patient rather like a menu. Instead, doctor and patient share ideas on what could be done, the pros and cons of various approaches and the acceptability of these approaches to patient and to doctor. Let us consider how this behaviour can be applied in a number of situations.

Firstly, engaging in this process when the initial management plan is discussed can prevent the concordance problems that are all too common.

A second example is the use of this behaviour when *difficulties* arise, when it can help with conflict resolution. For instance, imagine that an elderly patient did not comply with taking medication prescribed for hypertension. By thinking flexibly around the problem, we might establish that the patient did not agree with taking so many tablets, believing tablets to be a 'bad thing' (they have a point!). Our flexibility may be shown by our ability to discuss, explain and negotiate. As a result, the patient may agree to taking a smaller number of tablets, resulting in *some* reduction in blood pressure but perhaps not to target levels.

A third example is the application of this behaviour to non-clinical problems. For example, suppose a high DNA (did not attend) rate was found with a certain group of patients. One response could be to contact the patients and attempt to educate/discipline them about the appropriate use of services. However, with the mindset of ' thinking flexibly around problems' we may look at the characteristics of the group, inquire about the reasons for not attending and ask ourselves whether the problem might lie with the accessibility of doctor services rather than just with 'thoughtlessness' on the part of patients. Part of the solution might therefore be to alter the timing of some services.

No longer relies on rules alone but is able to use and justify discretionary judgement in situations of uncertainty.

This behaviour falls into the 'excellent' category, because it represents a high-order skill. For clarification, the first aspect of the behaviour 'no longer relies on rules alone' might suggest that good GPs should bend or break the rules. 'Rules' is a portmanteau word that could include guidelines as well as directives or instructions. The latter are rare, but examples include the procedures to be adopted under the mental health act or when referring for termination of pregnancy as well as clinical directives such as the pronouncements of the committee on safety of medicines.

Such rules should be followed, but guidelines are another matter. Nowadays, there are a plethora of guidelines and only a few are authoritative. We should understand the factors that differentiate good guidelines from the mediocre and in particular, should look to gauge the strength of evidence that underpins the guidelines and the composition of the group that formulated the advice. If the strength of evidence is weak, the guideline may hold little validity. If the composition the group suggests that the primary care has not been adequately represented, then the suggestions made may not be feasible or appropriate.

Good GPs will therefore move from simply *accepting* guidelines to *checking* for themselves through a process of critical thinking, whether the guidelines are appropriate or not. Let's now think about 'discretion' which means the freedom to judge or act on one's own.

Because uncertainty is one of the few certainties in general practice, there will be many situations in which guidelines are not available or applicable. This does not necessarily mean that *no* guidance is available. For example, the patient's problem may be similar but not identical to another problem for which advice is available and it might therefore be reasonable to extrapolate from one to the other. Therefore, although there may not be evidence from clinical trials to advise whether to use cholesterol-lowering drugs in the primary prevention of coronary heart disease in very elderly patients, we could make a good argument for active treatment.

In other situations, we may supplement our own opinion with that of an expert in a particular field, most commonly a hospital specialist. If such an opinion is not available or appropriate, we may rely upon our experience, in particular models or 'scripts' of how particular symptoms or problems have evolved in other patients. This may help us to recognise patterns as they emerge and also to anticipate what might happen in the near future.

For example, suppose a patient in his twenties presents with episodes of colicky abdominal pain. We might recognise features of irritable bowel syndrome but will also know that inflammatory bowel disease may present with similar symptoms at this age. We may use discretionary judgement to decide what near-patient tests to do and whether and when the patient needs to be referred for more invasive investigation.

Using discretionary judgement is vital for the expert GP and the 'watchful waiting' that GPs use, especially during the management of more complex problems, is an example of this skill in action.

In the next chapter, we will look at how the continuum of data-gathering and decision-making is used in its most frequent application in general practice, which is to our management of clinical problems.

9 Diagnostics: Clinical management

This performance area is about the recognition and management of common medical conditions in primary care.

In the previous two sections, data-gathering and making diagnoses/making decisions, we have learned about a number of behaviours that are needed to solve problems. These abilities are invaluable, because they can be applied to all problems, medical and non-medical, clinical and non-clinical and are particularly helpful for problems that, as in primary care, are more complex and don't have a single 'correct' solution.

In this chapter, we will move on and specifically apply these abilities to clinical problems that present in primary care.

Tip: learning from the curriculum

The GP curriculum describes elements of clinical management in the section 'primary care management'. Specifically, it advises:

Managing primary contact with patients, dealing with unselected problems requires:

- Knowledge of the epidemiology of problems presenting in primary care
- Mastering an approach that allows easy access for patients with unselected problems
- An organisational approach to the management of chronic conditions
- Knowledge of conditions encountered in primary care and their treatment.

Covering the full range of health conditions requires:

- Knowledge of preventative activities required in the practice of primary care
- Skills in acute, chronic, preventative, palliative and emergency care
- Clinical skills in history-taking, physical examination and use of ancillary tests to diagnose conditions presented by patients in primary care
- Skills in therapeutics, including drug and non-drug approaches to treatment of these conditions
- The ability to prioritise problems.

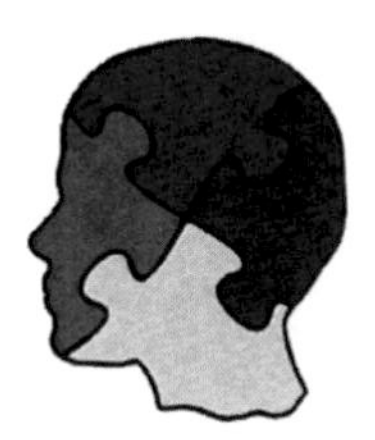

Joined up?
See p14

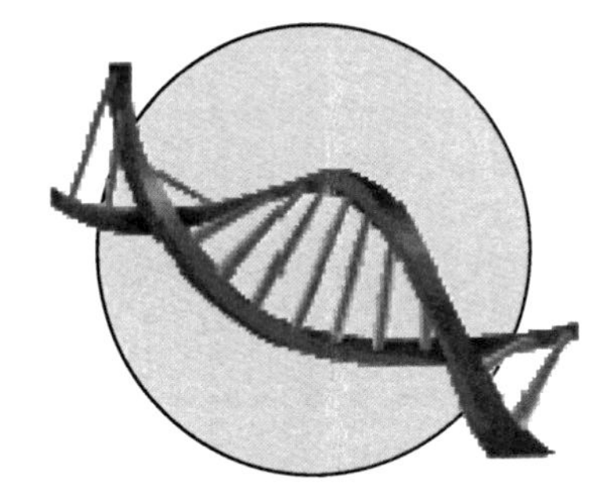

The behavioural traits that underpin 'clinical management' have been shown on page 60. This is a good time to refer back to them.

The 'clinical expertise' behaviours are needed particularly for the initial work-up of the clinical problem that then leads to a management plan being formulated. As we will see in this chapter, 'clinical management' also covers *referral*, for which empathy & sensitivity skills are needed when working with colleagues. It also covers the *follow-up* of the patient's problem whether it be a routine or emergency issue , including the provision of continuity of care. For this, the 'organisation skills' are particularly important. Such skills are also used in the related area of practice management and administration (see page 118). This illustrates how deeper features are generic because they are put to use in a variety of contexts.

There are seven major themes in the clinical management domain, each represented by a competency progression, which we will now discuss one by one:

Needs Further Development	Competent for licensing	Excellent	
Recognises the presentation of common physical, psychological and social problems.	Utilises the natural history of common problems in developing management plans.	Monitors the patient's progress to identify quickly unexpected deviations from the anticipated path.	1

This first progression is principally about learning to recognize the pattern of common problems. We move from:

Recognizing how common problems come to light in the community

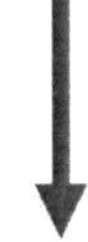

Understanding how these problems usually evolve and making use of this information to suggest appropriate treatment and follow-up plans

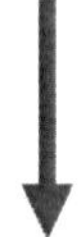

Ensuring, through advice and follow-up arrangements, that significant worsening or a failure to improve are brought to our attention.

Looking at each of the word pictures in turn:

Recognises the presentation of common physical, psychological and social problems.

This word picture refers to physical, psychological and social problems but should not be confused with 'holistic approach', where the competency is about being able to attend to these. Here, we are concerned with the ability to *recognise* common problems in these areas, particularly in the early stages. At the start of training, it's hard to know what is common and what isn't and this doesn't really become apparent until we are immersed in general practice. However, there are some ways that we can help ourselves (see box on the right)

What's common? Epidemiological data suggests that in rank order, the following types of disease tend to present most frequently. Note that the fifth most common condition in the community is a ragbag of ill-defined diseases, where no obvious pattern emerges.

1. Respiratory System diseases
2. Musculoskeletal Connective Tissue diseases
3. Skin & Subcutaneous Tissue diseases
4. Nervous System Sense organs diseases
5. Symptoms Signs of Ill defined diseases
6. Circulatory System diseases
7. Infectious Parasitic diseases

What's common in our locality?

In addition to knowing what the national figures suggest about prevalence, we also need to know how this translates to our local community. Getting to know our practice profile is important and the practice data manager can help to build up a picture of the types of patient in practice and in particular, how the profile differs from the fictional 'national average'.

For example, the age/sex profile of practices in Brighton (young people, young families) will be very different from Eastbourne (sometimes called Costa Geriatrica!). If our clientele are predominantly university students, we are very unlikely to become familiar with chronic disease management. Conversely, we are much more likely to have to manage eating disorders, so we should be on the lookout for them.

The locality may have pockets of patients with special needs, for example residential homes for the elderly, those with learning disabilities and with mental health problems.

Local employment and industry will influence the type of illnesses we deal with, so it helps to find out who the major employers are and (perhaps from the occupational health departments or local public health doctors) if there are any particular illnesses that we should be alert to. Employment rates are also a factor, with unemployment or changes in employment leading to psychological morbidity.

Tip: how can we learn to recognize common conditions?

Firstly, the curriculum identifies 'common and/or important conditions' in the clinical curriculum statements. This establishes the priorities and is a goldmine from which to develop our knowledge base.

Use techniques such as undertaking knowledge tests to find out where our gaps are and therefore our learning needs.

Keep a learning log of conditions that we are unsure of. What do these suggest about our patient's unmet needs and therefore our educational needs?

Learn to be curious. When seeing a patient, we should briefly look back over recent entries and identify how a condition first came to light. Also we should look at how the condition evolved as this can teach us about the natural history.

Local prevalence

What other factors can you think of that might affect the prevalence of disease and also the frequency of presentation?

Look at the data from your local commissioning group if you have one. Does this suggest any unusual characteristics about the practice that may relate to this issue?

Try sharing what you have learned with the practice team. This might stimulate interest as it is rare for doctors to a formally talk about this interesting topic.

With physical problems, what is the range of conditions we need to understand?

The curriculum describes the need for GPs to cover the 'full range of health conditions', which comprise:

- Skills in acute, chronic, preventative, palliative and emergency care
- Clinical skills in history taking, physical examination and use of ancillary tests to diagnose conditions presented in primary care
- Skills in therapeutics including drug and non-drug approaches to treatment of these conditions

In some areas, the ethnic profile may be associated with a different prevalence of certain conditions, such as CHD in diabetes in south Asians. In addition, the health beliefs and expectations of different cultures can vary considerably from the textbook norms.

This competency refers to common physical, social and psychological conditions. Therefore, we need to recognize common conditions in all three categories. What does 'common' mean? Here are some examples:

Physical:
Here are some examples of common and/or important conditions listed in the curriculum statement for the respiratory system:

- Upper respiratory tract infections: Sore throats and colds, tonsillitis, peri-tonsillar abscess, epiglottitis, laryngitis and tracheitis
- Lower respiratory tract infections: Influenza, bronchiolitis, bronchitis and pneumonia (of any cause)
- Acute non-infective respiratory problems: Allergy and anaphylaxis, hypersensitivity pneumonitis, pulmonary embolus, pneumothorax, aspiration of a foreign body
- Chronic lower respiratory problems: Chronic cough, asthma, chronic obstructive pulmonary disease (COPD), tuberculosis, cystic fibrosis, chronic interstitial lung diseases
- Lung cancer

Psychological:
The most common primary care mental health problems are depression, eating disorders, and anxiety disorders, ADHD, post-traumatic stress disorder, alcohol and drug misuse

Social:
Some situations, such as poverty, delinquency, unemployment, lack of adequate housing or care in the community are defined as social problems, whilst others, like white collar crime, fail to be classified in the same way and therefore attract little attention.
Interestingly, these problems are often defined in such a way that the focus is largely on the individual rather than the system. In general practice, many of the social problems that doctors deal with relate to relationship and behavioural difficulties and the fallout from these.

How is this indicator related to holistic practice?

Although we have given examples of physical, psychological & social problems under three separate headings, they don't usually occur separately in real life. As GPs, we need to be alert to the fact that problems in one of these areas tend to be associated with or to lead on to problems in the other two.

For example a young teenage boy with acne may attend for treatment. We may address the skin problem but then go on to explore the patient's feelings about his condition and ask about his mood. We could also ask about impact upon schooling. It might transpire that the patient is being harassed at school and has been truanting as a result. This simple example shows how the domains should not be thought of in isolation of each other. They are connected. The same boy could have been brought in by his parents with emotional distress or have been brought with the social problem of truanting. Careful enquiry would then have revealed the skin condition to be a significant common factor.

Looking at patients' problems in this way is an example of holistic practice, which is one of the expert skills of GPs. This approach helps us to identify significant problems that are related to each other and deal with them appropriately. It also helps us to anticipate and prevent a problem in another domain, before it occurs. For instance, dealing effectively with acne may reduce the chances of depression in the adolescent and possibly the chances of being bullied.

Significant or serious conditions often start out masquerading as common or minor ones. For example, Polymyalgia may in the early stages be diagnosed as arthritis. Hyporthyroidism may initially be thought to be post-viral fatigue. Most if not all significant conditions have, especially in the early stages, a differential diagnosis that includes common disorders.

Therefore, knowing about common conditions is important if we are to diagnose serious ones. This is because knowing how common conditions develop and resolve helps us to recognise when the patient's problem is beginning to fall outside this pattern.

Red flags

We looked at the importance of red flags in the previous section 'making diagnoses' (see page 72). It is vital to think about common symptoms like headache, dizziness, back pain and indigestion.

What are the serious conditions and their red flag symptoms and signs that you should check for in relation to each of these?

There are national guidelines for many common symptoms that will help you to answer this question.

Utilises the natural history of common problems in developing management plans.

Having recognized what we think is a common condition, the next step is to think about the differential diagnosis and ask whether there are any significant or serious conditions with which the common condition might be confused. Asking about the red flag symptoms or signs of serious disease can be vital. Although it may feel like a tedious exercise, thinking of a common condition as being a 'diagnosis of exclusion' can keep our actions safe.

For example in a middle-aged man with a two week history of a hoarse voice, a diagnosis of a viral infection may be made. In the course of reaching this diagnosis and devising a management plan, we might investigate the differential diagnosis by asking about dysphagia (oesophageal cancer), cigarette smoking (laryngeal pathology) and asthma (oral thrush from the use of steroid inhaler). If the answers are negative, we can use our knowledge of viral laryngeal infections to decide the appropriate follow-up period. In this example, the patient might be asked to return if symptoms are still persisting after a further two weeks.

Improving our understanding of natural history

From the records, look back on the management of common conditions such as respiratory and musculoskeletal problems. Some problems will be acute and self-limiting and from these we can learn the time taken for the condition to reach its peak and then resolve.

Other conditions, such as arthritis, are chronic. We may learn many things about the natural history such as how commonly exacerbations occur, which joints are most affected, factors that exacerbate or relieve the condition and how patients fare when managed in different ways, including using their own remedies. Information about these factors can help us to formulate appropriate management plans, for example advising whether medication might help or not.

Assessor's corner

For assessors, looking at the follow up plans that doctors make is a quick way of telling whether the doctor's understanding of natural history is sound.

This understanding can also be probed directly in case-based discussions.

Understanding the natural history also helps us to judge whether treatment is essential, desirable, optional, unnecessary or potentially harmful. For example, many symptoms such as coryza are within normal experience and therefore do not need to be medicalised.

Explanation about the natural history is important in demedicalising symptoms and also helps patients to understand the management plan, the safety net and what actions they might take. For example when to get a deferred prescription dispensed, contact a doctor, go to hospital or return to the GP if their progress is not as good as expected.

Monitors the patient's progress to identify quickly unexpected deviations from the anticipated path.

Unlike in secondary care, where we exclude more serious disease through a large number of tests performed at one point in time, in primary care we exclude by collecting information through tests and observation over a period of time, looking for deviations from an expected path of recovery.

We could say that time is the GPs 'MRI scan'.

This competency is about the management and follow-up plans that we make, rather than our clinical skills per se. Earlier on, we talked about the deeper features. The organisation and planning abilities are the most relevant to this area of performance and we use them to think ahead and construct appropriate safety nets. Safety nets, like all nets, have holes. It is therefore important, for any given problem, not to rely on one net but to put in place a number that between them can reduce the chance of a serious problem slipping through without being caught.

The follow-up arrangements should allow serious conditions to be identified and acted upon early enough to avoid putting the patient at undue risk.

For example, suppose a college student presents with migraine headaches having not had any for some time. The clinical assessment reveals associated nausea and mild photophobia, but no other positive findings. Although migraine is possible, indeed probable, there is a risk of meningitis especially in the student group and the patient may be asked to return shortly to check that no new and suspicious findings are present.

It is through such reviews that we learn more about the natural history of the problem, the likelihood of other conditions being present and the evolution of more serious conditions. This information helps us to make better decisions and improve our management plans.

'Monitoring the patient's progress' is not entirely a doctor-based activity and is increasingly undertaken by the team.

Good record keeping in which our thoughts are made clear is a vital part of ensuring that other health professionals understand our thoughts on what the 'anticipated path' is and therefore recognise when unexpected deviations occur. To reduce risk to patients even further, it can be really helpful to record our thoughts as to *what may need to be done* if deviations occur. For example, a GP treating a patient with chronic cough may write 'consider chest x-ray if symptoms not cleared within the next two weeks'. Sometimes, doctors can be reticent to write in this way, particularly when they are training, inexperienced, are not regular members of the practice team or are worried that their thoughts might make them look foolish. That would be a shame because it's the thoughts that flow from the patient encounter that are often more valuable than the record of the encounter itself.

So far, we have talked in terms of acute conditions, but this competency also applies to the management of chronic conditions. For these, there will usually need to be more systematic surveillance accompanied by a programme of patient education and support. Coronary heart disease is a good example in which we see doctors orchestrating management as a team-based activity, involving the patient and family.

For coronary disease, an example of an 'unexpected deviation' may be an exacerbation of chest pain or breathlessness which occurs without warning and may suggest an acute event. We might construct a safety net for the patient without knowing whether and when it might be used but for coronary disease such a net might include education, information leaflets, an emergency supply of GTN and instructions on the circumstances in which an ambulance should be called.

Needs Further Development	Competent for licensing	Excellent
Responds to the problem by routinely suggesting intervention.	Considers simple therapy/ expectant measures where appropriate.	Uses drug and non-drug methods in the treatment of the patient, appropriately using traditional and complementary medical approaches.

2

Having recognized the problem, this progression describes how we change from an interventionist approach (common and important in secondary care) to an approach that uses conventional treatment (drug and non-drug), complementary therapy and where appropriate, no treatment at all.

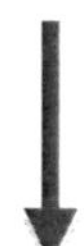

We recognise a problem, but instead of (where appropriate) watching and waiting to see how the condition evolves, we take action and intervene, for example with a prescription or a referral.

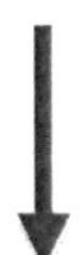

In addition to being able to recommend when to watch and wait, we are also able to recommend simple remedies and self-help and monitor the situation rather than intervene.

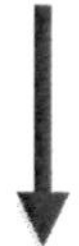

We are able to think of 'treatment' in a broad sense and are able to accept non-drug and complementary approaches and recommend them appropriately.

Looking at each of the word pictures in turn:

Responds to the problem by routinely suggesting intervention.

Doctors who are relatively inexperienced in primary care tend to respond in this way. This is not surprising, because in the hospital context it is not appropriate to 'watch and wait' as the job of the hospital specialist is to banish uncertainty by gathering data and taking action. In primary care, patient problems are unfiltered, presenting to us without having first being assessed by another doctor. It's quite possible that the problem with which the patient presents isn't actually 'medical' or amenable to a doctor's skills. Part of our skill is being able to recognise when this might be the case.

'Intervention' means taking some form of direct action that might include ordering tests and investigations, referring a patient or recommending treatment.

Considers simple therapy/expectant measures where appropriate.

If we are unable to do anything more than routinely intervene (do tests/ prescribe/refer), this means that we have not yet learned that in primary care, problems often need to be given time to evolve and become discernible before appropriate intervention can be recommended. During the waiting phase, it may well be appropriate to suggest simple measures (e.g. cough linctus) whilst we are waiting to see whether the condition resolves as expected.

In addition to medication and simple remedies, a broader palette of options is needed in primary care partly because many problems will not have a satisfactory ' traditional' medical solution. There may not be a 'pill for every ill' and many ills need no treatment at all.

Part of this competency therefore, is knowing when *not* to prescribe, for example when not to give antibiotics for a cough. To be effective, this ability needs to be linked with good communication skills so that the patient understands the pros and cons of treatment and is able to accept the recommendation not to treat.

Simple treatments include traditional remedies such as steam inhalation, basic medications such as painkillers and over-the-counter (OTC) preparations. The latter used to be mainly simple (i.e. not prescription-only) medications but with changes to prescribing regulations and the community pharmacists role, this is no longer the case and an increasing number of complex preparations are available without a doctor consultation. It is therefore increasingly important to check what OTC drugs the patient may have taken.

'Considering simple therapy' also includes trying to recommend the simplest of the appropriate options. For example, there may be no need for strong painkillers or combination therapies when a less potent drug or a single medication would do.

Simple treatments are not a separate class of management but are often an initial part of a management process that might later lead on to a higher degree of medical intervention. For example, patients with dyspepsia may begin with OTC antacids but later move on to acid- suppression, breath testing and possible gastroscopy. Note that nowadays most of the steps in this example of a continuum of simple to complex measures, can be implemented by or with the pharmacist, which is an example of their enhanced role.

Uses drug and non-drug methods in the treatment of the patient, appropriately using traditional and complementary medical approaches.

In primary care, many forms of help are available. These may include giving explanations, using non-drug interventions such as lifestyle advice or physiotherapy and where appropriate, supporting the patient in the use of complementary therapy. With the latter it may be that doctors do not make a formal recommendation or referral, but that where the patient wishes to go down this route and harm is unlikely, we do not stand in the way and may even facilitate this action.

Needs Further Development	Competent for licensing	Excellent
Uses appropriate but limited management options with little flexibility for the preferences of others.	Varies management options responsively according to the circumstances, priorities and preferences of those involved.	Generates and offers justifiable approaches where specific guidelines are not available.

3

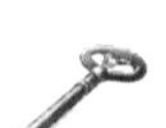

For many educators, this is a particularly important progression in the domain of clinical management. In particular, the 'competent' descriptor is significant as we shall describe later.

This progression describes how we start off with a safe but limited and relatively rigid range of options, become more flexible and responsive with an increasing range of approaches and finally, create new approaches where alternatives are not available.

We move from:

Initially having only a limited range of options, although making use of these appropriately. The narrowness of these options means that we have little choice on offer, which in turn makes us less flexible and adaptable to what the patient wants.

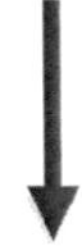

Building up, through experience, a wider range of management options which when coupled with the wish to be flexible, allows us to respond to what the patient needs.

Being able to think for ourselves and suggest approaches that are *tailored* to the situation. Although these approaches may not have an explicit evidence-based, perhaps because there are no guidelines that directly address the problem, they can still be justified.

Looking at each of the word pictures in turn:

Uses appropriate but limited management options with little flexibility for the preferences of others.

This progression is interesting because it is partly about acting *appropriately* but also about being able to *tailor* plans, modifying them in response to the thoughts of others, in particular the patient.

You may think that the knowledge and skill base of the GP is fairly standard stuff and will come through experience. This may be the case, but we have to remember that primary care is different from what we have experienced in secondary care. Patients come with *problems* rather than symptoms or signs, which means that we first have to clarify the problem, remembering to think of social and psychological problems as well as clinical ones.

Additionally, we have to tailor our plans. Look at the box on the left to read why this is important. Tailored plans are like tailored (rather than 'off the peg') suits. Patients feel much more comfortable in them and are more likely to wear them and come back to the tailor when the next plan needs designing!

In addition to our clinical abilities, the other major feature of this competency is the *interest* that we take in the patient and the desire we have to respond to their needs. To continue with the clothing analogy, in order to produce a custom-made suit, we have to know the patient's measurements; in other words we have to be interested enough to know what the patient's *requirements* are.

At the 'NFD' level we show little flexibility for patient's needs and this can be due to a number of reasons:

- Firstly, we may not *know enough* to be able to adapt our plans even if we wanted to. Doctors often take refuge in being rigid (for example sticking to their plans and telling patients what to do) when they can't think of suitable alternatives.
- Secondly, we may simply not see the value of tailoring plans or of being flexible. In other words, even if we have the skills to offer a range of options, we may not have the right *attitude.*
- Thirdly, we may not have the *skills to negotiate* a plan with the patient. Tailoring is not the same as just doing what the patient wants, and negotiation skills are needed when there might be conflict.

If you have difficulty with this competency, ask yourself whether the problem lies with your clinical skills, your attitude, your communication (especially negotiation) skills or a combination of these.

These areas work in synergy, which means that improving any one of them will improve the whole. For example, if you have better clinical skills you will feel more confident in offering a wider range of options and this will improve your attitude to being flexible with patients. Here's an interesting point; even if you feel that you don't have many options to offer, if you have the attitude of sharing the plan with the patient, *they* are likely to generate suitable options that had not occurred to you. To use a cliché, the patient is part of the solution as well as part of the problem!

Varies management options responsively according to the circumstances, priorities and preferences of those involved.

Why do educators consider this to be such an important competency? The reason is that it embodies the observation and responsiveness that GPs need to show in their clinical practice.

Question: Why is the ability to tailor plans important?

The ability to tailor plans rather than seek to impose an inflexible option means that plans are much more likely to be followed.

Because concordance is improved, **treatment** is likely to be more effective, **waste** (from for example unused medication or non-attendance at hospital appointments) is reduced and the **adverse consequences** of less appropriate treatment, avoided. Can you see how the ability to tailor plans is therefore linked with good risk management?

Importantly, tailored plans show that we have *interest* and *respect* for the patient's thoughts and preferences. This improves trust and the doctor-patient relationship generally, which itself makes future plans easier to negotiate. This can be vital when the plan concerns a problem in which uncertainty or the risk of conflict are significant.

In the same way as we must not assume that our initial working diagnosis is the right one, we must also not assume that the initial management plan will remain the best one as time goes on.

We need to continually look at how well the plan is working from both our own and the patient's perspective, checking out whether other options become important as the situation changes and therefore whether the plan needs to change.

Generates and offers justifiable approaches where specific guidelines are not available.

Compared to 'NFD', at the 'competent' level we still produce appropriate management options but the menu of possible choices that we generate and offer becomes much broader.

This competency overlaps with the ones listed below, which come from the performance area of 'Making a diagnosis/making decisions':

- *Thinks flexibly around problems, generating functional solutions.*
- *No longer relies on rules alone but is able to use and justify discretionary judgement in situations of uncertainty.*

It is worth re-reading the explanation of these competencies from page 76.

The current competency refers to being able to generate approaches when guidelines are not available. It is not about the quality and legitimacy of the guidelines (which are covered in the Making a diagnosis/making decisions') but about our mindset.

At this level of performance, we have moved beyond tailoring existing guidance and are able to be creative when no recommended option seems to be available from the books or guidelines. Of course, this does not mean that we are allowed to behave idiosyncratically. Whatever approaches we suggest must be justifiable on the basis of accepted medical practice. 'Generating' the approach does not necessarily mean that we have to come up with an original suggestion. In real life, we don't wait for inspiration but we usually discuss the case with GP colleagues or hospital specialists, whose thoughts may prompt new ideas.

Question: In what way is 'generating approaches' related to risk management?

This competency takes us and our patients into uncertain territory. By definition, a recommended approach is not available, which means that we must evaluate the risk associated with the approaches that are generated. This requires a good deal of experience with risk management and, preferably, experience with this type of problem; the latter is not always available. It also requires considerable expertise with communication skills.

For example, we may need to explain the situation, the degree of uncertainty and the possible risks of using an approach that may be a modification of an existing approach, or something entirely new.

Care needs to be taken not to simply accept the patient's willingness to put their trust in us, but to try to explain so that the patient can make an informed choice. We also need to be careful not to *insist* upon an informed choice if the patient (or their advocate) is unwilling or unable to engage in the process.

Varying plans responsively

It is common for doctors to suggest changes to the plan, but much less common for patients to be asked without first being made aware of the doctor's thoughts.

We will often have clinical reasons for suggesting changes, but (because we are not the patient) we won't know the impact that the plan is having on the patient's life. This is a vital piece in the jigsaw.

Try asking patients how things are going and how, if at all, they wish to modify the plan *before* you make suggestions of your own.

Needs Further Development	Competent for licensing	Excellent
Makes appropriate prescribing decisions, routinely using important sources of information.	Routinely checks on drug interactions and side effects and shows awareness of national and local prescribing guidance.	Prescribes cost-effectively but is able to justify transgressions of this principle.

4

This indicator is specifically concerned with prescribing and describes how we move from:

Prescribing safely, using appropriate sources of information and doing so routinely and dependably, rather than occasionally and inconsistently.

Prescribing in accordance with guidelines, protocols and computer prompts. Establishing which side-effects and interactions might occur and routinely checking for the presence or absence of these with the patient.

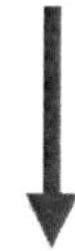

Being aware of cost issues, seeking to prescribe the most cost-effective of the available and appropriate alternatives. Being prepared to prescribe less frugally, or outside the formulary, when appropriate.

Looking at each of the word pictures in turn:

Makes appropriate prescribing decisions, routinely using important sources of information.

The key behaviour in this indicator is our routine use of guidance. *Why is this important?* In other areas of clinical performance such as the knowledge of appropriate investigations and the patterns that may suggest particular diagnoses, the knowledge base is relatively stable and the mechanisms of CPD are usually adequate to maintain safe practice.

However, with prescribing, changes occur much more frequently and the effects of 'getting it wrong' through side-effects, interactions and the wrong choice of drug can be more immediate, profound and sometimes dangerous. Because of the range of drugs and their associated features and the multiple combinations of medication, we need to be in the habit of *not* relying on our memories when prescribing as much as we do for other areas of clinical care.

The important sources of information in general practice are textbooks such as the British National formulary, whether in paper form or online, and the numerous computer prompts on practice systems that warn of side-effects, significant drug interactions and recommended drug options. Doctors who are not competent tend to either fail to check on appropriate prescribing options, to disregard prompts or both. Even if their prescribing is safe to begin with, such behaviour will result over a fairly short timescale, in unsafe practice.

Routinely checks on drug interactions and side effects and shows awareness of national and local prescribing guidance.

This competency refers to the habit of checking the literature to decide on which drug to prescribe and this leads us on to the next competency.

It takes the previous one forward in two ways:

- Firstly we not only use the literature to decide what to prescribe but also, when initiating medication and when following up the patient, we discuss side-effects and check on interactions. Checking is important because adverse effects may take time to show themselves, for example the dry cough with ACEI or muscle pain with statins. Very often, patients find the information sheets that come with their drugs overwhelming and frightening. As a result, they often rely on doctors to advise on important interactions.

- Secondly, we go beyond checking on individual drugs and pay heed to national guidelines, often related to particular conditions such as asthma, and to local prescribing guidance such as the practice formulary.

Prescribes cost-effectively but is able to justify transgressions of this principle.

Prescribing cost-effectively is clearly important because of the finite resources of the health service and the opportunity-costs that inefficient prescribing creates. There are many measures that we can take to keep costs down, including prescribing generically wherever appropriate (it isn't always), prescribing from a limited list of cost-effective drugs, establishing patient preferences so that prescribed medication is likely to be taken and managing repeat prescriptions to prevent stockpiling and wastage.

Question: what factors might influence the management plan?

First and foremost, the ideas, concerns and expectations of the patient could have a direct bearing. These will determine the patient's preferences for what should be done and will help us to suggest which option, from a list of appropriate alternatives, might best fit these preferences.

We need empathy and sensitivity to take an interest in the patient's perspective, coupled with good communication skills to elicit the patient's preferences.

We also have our own priorities and these should be shared as they may result in the patient modifying their own preferences until an accommodation is reached. This process is at the heart of negotiation.

Beyond doctor and patient, there are other factors that may influence the plan. On the patient's side, the priorities and preferences of significant people such as family or employers may modify the patient's thinking.

On our side, beyond the clinical assessment our preferences may be influenced by the availability of resources, the direction given by guidelines and personal factors such as personal biases formed by previous clinical experiences.

Question: When might you knowingly prescribe less cost-effectively?

The main aim is not to keep costs to a minimum but to keep *cost-effectiveness* to a maximum. It is pointless using cheap drugs if they do not treat the patient's problem or are in some way unacceptable to the patient. Good GPs move from being a doctor-centred to being appropriately patient-centred. Therefore, the most common reason for prescribing less cost-effectively is because this is the best way of addressing the patient's needs. For example, the patient may have a preference for a particular formulation, such as paracetamol capsules rather than tablets. They may have co morbidity such as dyspepsia, which may make an enteric-coated preparation preferable.

The drug may have to fit in with a *lifestyle* choice, such as when gelatin-free products are needed for vegetarians and vegans. Occasionally, patients may not be happy with taking tablets several times a day when a modified - release preparation is available, as for example with diclofenac. Similarly, patients may hear of combination preparations that they would prefer to separate items.

Another issue is the variability between generic preparations of the same drug. Often, being dispensed drugs that are the same but look different is merely an inconvenience. However, when it causes confusion, there may be risk attached. Occasionally, patients are adamant that some generic preparations cause side-effects when compared to others and there may then be a case for prescribing a trade name to guarantee consistency in what the patient receives.

Nowadays, when faced with situations such as those described, it is not unreasonable for doctors to discuss the need for cost containment with patients. Many patients are willing to help the NHS to save money when this is possible, but it is our duty to weigh up the risks and benefits of doing so. Balancing this is the realisation that patient choice matters: there is no more expensive drug than one that isn't taken!

Needs Further Development	Competent for licensing	Excellent	
Performs up to, but does not exceed, the limits of their own competence.	Refers appropriately and co-ordinates care with other professionals in primary care and with other specialists.	Identifies and encourages the development of new resources where these are needed.	**5**

This progression concerns our ability to make use of and then improve the help that is available to our patients. We move from:

Being able and willing to use our personal abilities to the fullest, in the interests of the patient, whilst not going beyond what we are capable of.

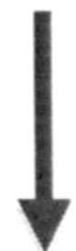

Bringing in and coordinating other resources, particularly other healthcare workers to assist in the management of the patient's problem.

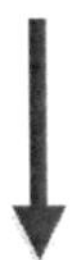

Recognizing gaps in the primary care service and addressing these when they are significant.

Looking at each of the word pictures in turn:

Performs up to, but does not exceed, the limits of their own competence.

This competency involves two significant elements. Firstly, we have to be willing to accept responsibility for 'doing the job' i.e. not leaving things undone or passing the buck inappropriately. Secondly, we need a reliable system for checking our own competence.

Question: How could you check that you are not exceeding your limit of competence?

Firstly, this can be done by reflecting on your actions and their outcomes. Prospectively, a log diary of situations in which you were *uncertain* will allow you to look back on the outcomes and decide whether your management was appropriate. Keeping a record of *referrals* will help you to gauge the frequency of referral to different specialties and whether these indicate over- or under-referral. It will help you to gauge appropriateness in terms of whether more could have been done to investigate the problem before referral, whether the appropriate specialty was chosen and whether the advice or intervention the hospital provided could have been offered by a GP.

Secondly, to develop insight into performance, comparisons need to be made, particularly against actions of competent colleagues with whom you work. Talking through cases and looking at how others deal with similar problems can help you to do this. In parallel with this, the competence framework of the MRCGP allows you to make comparisons with the national standards described.

Thirdly, feedback from colleagues is invaluable and this can either be informal through case review or formalised through structured assessments. Powerful but less palatable feedback comes from significant events and complaints, which may indicate areas in which you may *not have done* certain things that a competent doctor should have done or in which you have gone beyond your competence by *doing certain things* that you may not have had the judgement or skills to do.

The mechanisms of checking our competence, described in the box are invaluable and may confirm that we are acting within our limits. However, acting within the *comfort zone* may not be good enough if our limits do not extend as far as needed for a competent GP. Checking on competence may flag up areas of under-performance that may need addressing, with significant events and patient safety issues being examples that may require urgent attention.

Refers appropriately and co-ordinates care with other professionals in primary care and with other specialists.

In this competency, we move beyond being reliant upon our own skills and make use of other health professionals within the primary health care team and from secondary care. In addition to referral, we *coordinate* the activities of those to whom we refer by:

- *Monitoring* who is doing what, keeping individuals informed of what they need to know
- *Reviewing* the patient periodically to gauge response to treatment
- Looking for *evolution* of the patient's condition
- Modifying management, safety netting and monitoring for the unexpected.

Unfortunately, good communication with the patient is not as widespread in some branches of the health service as it is in primary care. This needs to change and an important part of the GPs review of the patient is to *explain* what has happened and what has been found by other professionals and to *check* the patient's understanding and elicit their concerns.

Identifies and encourages the development of new resources where these are needed.

This competency is in the excellent category and is not a skill that we usually have the opportunity to demonstrate. It overlaps with 'community orientation' and it is worth reading the section on page 135.

It is a continuation of the GP mindset of looking for ways in which to help manage the patient's problem. Sometimes, doctors identify a patient need, but find that either a resource to meet the need does not exist, or else that it exists but is not accessible. For example, patients with suspected heart failure cannot be adequately diagnosed on clinical grounds alone. Usually, an echocardiogram is needed and in some regions, this investigation is directly accessible by GPs, preventing significant delays that might have an adverse effect on the patient's health.

Using this example, a doctor who performs at this level might act as patient-advocate for both the individual and for his community of patients by campaigning for the provision of an open-access echocardiogram service. Nowadays, there are mechanisms for GPs to have a direct influence on service provision in the locality through commissioning processes.

Needs Further Development	Competent for licensing	Excellent
Ensures that continuity of care can be provided for the patient's problem e.g. through adequate record keeping.	Provides continuity of care for the patient rather than just the problem, reviewing care at suitable intervals.	Contributes to an organisational infrastructure and professional culture that allows continuity of care to be facilitated and valued.

6

Having dealt with the ways in which we can provide help for the patient by using our own skill and by involving others, this progression illustrates the importance of providing personal continuity of care. We move from:

Ensuring that those who follow us in managing the patient's problem are adequately informed, particularly through good record keeping.

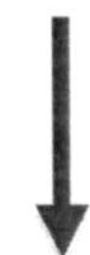

Taking steps to personally review the patient, keeping an overview of their health, an interest in their thoughts and experience and developing an understanding of the patient as a *person*.

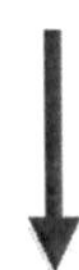

Modifying attitudes and the working environment so that continuity of care can be understood, valued and made the best use of.

Looking at each of the word pictures in turn:

Ensures that continuity of care can be provided for the patient's problem e.g. through adequate record keeping.

Continuity of care is highly valued by GPs and patients, but why is it considered worthwhile? The interest and responsibility we take in the patient's health over a significant period of time helps us to develop a relationship of trust. This allows for more open and honest communication, more concordant management plans and therefore a more effective use of medical time in optimising the patient's health.

Additionally, the relationship of trust means that there is greater tolerance and flexibility on both sides. This is important because virtually all patients develop significant conditions at some time in their lives and most such conditions have innocuous beginnings, which can be misdiagnosed as minor ailments. In a trusting relationship, doctors may be less *fearful* of (although they should be no less *alert* for) situations where the patient's problem is evolving in a way that was not expected. Where the nature of the problem or the best management plan are unclear, if we have the patient's trust we may be more willing to watch and wait or use our professional judgement. In effect, having trust means that patients are more willing to accept short-term risks that may mean that over-investigation, over-treatment or inappropriate referral are avoided.

Continuity of care also means that we can tailor plans better because we understand how the patient's mind and body are likely to respond. For the same reason of trust, the patient is more likely to concord with a plan and to be more tolerant and forgiving when things go wrong.

Lastly, continuity of care means that we are better able to understand the patient's context, which includes their family, and thereby support them better. At this basic level of competence, we have to demonstrate that we can provide continuity of care for the patient's problem throughout record-keeping and follow-up arrangements.

Question: How might record-keeping assist continuity of care?

Notes can assist continuity of care by recording the basics (history, examination, investigation) and also the patient's thoughts, preferences and responses.

They also record our own thoughts including working diagnosis, management plan, safety netting and anticipatory thinking (thinking ahead).

Coding the diagnoses and significant problems is particularly important as this allows stages of a particular journey to be electronically linked, presented and understood. This also improves patient safety.

Our management plan and anticipatory thinking are at their best when they suggest to a third party what response to management we were looking for, when and by whom the patient should be followed up and what we were planning to do next time.

This ensures that the richness of information gained from dialogue with the patient is not lost, the danger being that if it is not recorded, not only can it not be used but it may not be *elicited* again.

Provides continuity of care for the patient rather than just the problem, reviewing care at suitable intervals.

In this competency, we move beyond good *technical* medicine and no longer see the patient in terms of their problem, but as a *person.*

The competent GP is proactive with follow-up arrangements and rather than leave the patient to make an unguided choice (or worse, regularly advise the patient to see some other doctor), encourages the patient to return to him or her. This does not mean that we should review every problem, as this would be unnecessary and impossible. However, there are ways in which we can maintain the thread of continuity over the years with the patient. For example, we might follow through significant problems with which we are involved. We might also encourage the patient to come back to us for routine medication reviews at which time we could briefly look through significant problems in the records with which other doctors have been involved.

The opportunities to undertake medication reviews are becoming less as nurses take over some of these duties, particularly in chronic disease management. This might mean that we have to make greater use of opportunistic situations to update ourselves on the patient's story, for example on home visits. Of course there are some situations in which all doctors would try to provide personal continuity, most notably with palliative care.

Contributes to an organisational infrastructure and professional culture that allows continuity of care to be facilitated and valued.

As with many of the 'excellent' competencies, this is difficult to achieve for doctors who are only members of the practice team for a relatively short time. Nevertheless, it is possible for doctors in training to show that they value continuity of care and to make it easier for others to engage with this. For example, trainees can keep the 'usual doctor' updated when they have been involved in a patient's care, particularly about significant issues. This can be done easily through conversation or by leaving a paper or electronic note. Additionally, trainees can keep the sort of medical records that encourage continuity as described in the box on the left.

Acting in these ways are practical examples of how continuity of care can be facilitated.

Needs Further Development	Competent for licensing	Excellent
Responds rapidly and skilfully to emergencies.	Appropriately follows-up patients who have experienced a medical emergency, and their family.	Ensures that emergency care is co-ordinated within the practice team and integrated with the emergency services.

7

This progression is specifically about one aspect of clinical management, namely dealing with emergencies. We move from:

Being competent in handling emergency situations in primary care

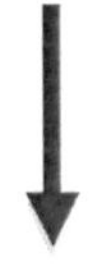

Being able to deal with the aftermath of an emergency both with the patient and with their family

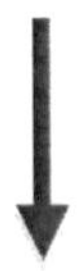

Ensuring that emergency care is a coordinated team-based activity

Looking at each of the word pictures in turn:

Responds rapidly and skilfully to emergencies.

The out-of-hours competency framework covers the skills required to meet this behaviour. We need to be biomedically competent with dealing with emergencies ranging from CPR to psychiatric emergencies. We also need to be adequately prepared, including having the requisite equipment and drugs, which are replenished and kept in date.

Emergency care is stressful and our reactions should be appropriate and proportionate, so that medical conditions that are less serious are not admitted as emergencies and conditions that are true emergencies are recognised.

In addition, we should be able to use the appropriate emergency services including domiciliary emergency care workers, 'Hospital at home' services, social services, psychiatric crisis teams and so on. We should also be capable of keeping others (and ourselves) calm in a crisis. This is difficult, but comes with experience.

Tip: emergency care

With some emergencies, in particular cardio-respiratory collapse, regular training and occasional drills are needed so that in a real emergency, very little 'thinking' is required by those involved because the necessary actions have become reflex.

This is important because thinking under pressure is difficult and is easy to get wrong because of the emotions involved.

Appropriately follows-up patients who have experienced a medical emergency, and their family.

Part of our holistic mindset is to consider the wider context and in particular, the impact of an emergency on the patients life, work, relationships and family members. An emergency will be a significant event in these peoples' lives and following-up the emergency has a number of functions including talking it through, hearing thoughts, identifying concerns and providing information and education. We can help the patient to understand what happened, what the implications are and what to do in the event of a future emergency. As a by-product, this also can reduce the likelihood of complaint, whether on not complaint was justified.

It may be that treatment changes have been made or further investigations are planned and part of the follow-up is to ensure that the required changes have been carried through.

Following-up the patient is also an example of maintaining continuity of care and supporting the patient and family at a difficult time. Emergencies are usually significant events for the medical professionals involved and lessons can be learned from informal reflection or formal significant event meetings. The latter can help to ascertain whether the emergency could have been avoided or anticipated (perhaps through better clinical management or patient education) and whether any practice training needs have been flagged up, such as CPR training or how to deal with a confused and aggressive patient.

Ensures that emergency care is co-ordinated within the practice team and integrated with the emergency services.

This competency requires doctors to think about emergency care as a team-based activity. Emergencies may be primarily physical, psychological or social. For example, the team might respond to a collapse in surgery, a patient who telephones in a suicidal state or a bruised child who might be a victim of physical abuse. Each of these problems requires coordinated activity so that drama is kept to a minimum, urgent attention is given, confidentiality and dignity are preserved and 'normal service' to other patients is maintained as far as possible.

Integration with emergency services requires the team to have knowledge of who or what is the appropriate service to contact, to learn from the outcomes of emergencies and modify the future use of emergency services where required.

We have now covered the process of decision-making and looked in detail at the various facets of clinical management. As we become proficient with these areas, it becomes possible to grapple with the hardest area of all, 'managing medical complexity' which is described in the following chapter.

10 Diagnostics: Managing medical complexity

This performance area is about aspects of care beyond managing straightforward problems, including the management of co-morbidity, uncertainty and risk, and the approach to health rather than just illness.

In the previous three sections of 'diagnostics' we have learned the theory of decision-making through data-gathering & making diagnoses/making decisions. We have then gone on to apply these skills to the primary care context in 'clinical management'.

In the final section on 'diagnostics', we move beyond the straightforward problems described in clinical management and look at some of the difficult areas where GP expertise comes into its own. It takes years of experience to master the competencies described here, but a basic ability to understand the concepts and apply them is required for licensing. The reason is that if the competencies are not there in rudimentary form, there is no foundation on which to build this vital area of expertise.

Learning from the curriculum

The GP curriculum describes the elements of 'managing medical complexity' in the section '*comprehensive approach*'

Simultaneously managing multiple complaints and pathologies, both acute and chronic health problems requires:

- An understanding of the concept of co-morbidity in a patient
- The skill to manage the concurrent health problems experienced by a patient through identification, exploration, negotiation, acceptance and prioritisation
- The *skill* to seek, and the *attitude* to use, the best evidence in practice

Promoting health and wellbeing by applying health promotion and disease prevention strategies appropriately requires:

- The ability to understand the concept of health
- The ability to promote health on an individual basis as part of the consultation
- The ability to promote health through a health promotion or disease prevention programme within the primary care setting
- Understanding the role of the GP in health promotion activities in the community
- Understanding and recognising the importance of ethical tensions between the needs of the individual and the community, and acting appropriately.

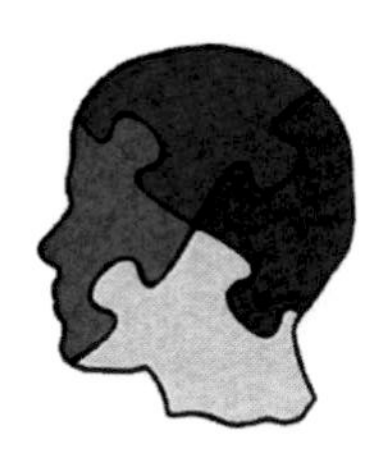

Joined up?
See p14

Managing and coordinating health promotion, prevention, cure, care, rehabilitation and palliation requires:

- Understanding the complex nature of health problems in general practice
- Understanding the variety of possible approaches
- The ability to use different approaches in an individual patient and to modify these according to an individual's needs
- The ability to coordinate teamwork in primary care

This section more than any other in the competence framework, describes the particular expertise of GPs. In many proposed health service reforms, particularly those in which GPs lose continuity of care with a registered list of their own patients, 'medical complexity' is at risk. This may result in:

- An inability to manage the list of problems with which patients often come, which can lead to lack of appropriate prioritisation based on risk. In addition, the patient's main agenda item may not be recognised. This may lead to patient dissatisfaction, higher consultation rates and increased work-related stress.
- An inability to effectively promote health, which means that patients are not sufficiently encouraged or educated in how to take some responsibility for their own health. Patients therefore become less effective partners in keeping their side of the bargain in a shared management plan.
- Lack of health promotion interventions means that there may be additional treatment costs for conditions that should have been prevented.
- If doctors do not show a sustained and positive attitude to a patient's health, there may also be slower recovery rates for those patients are already under treatment.

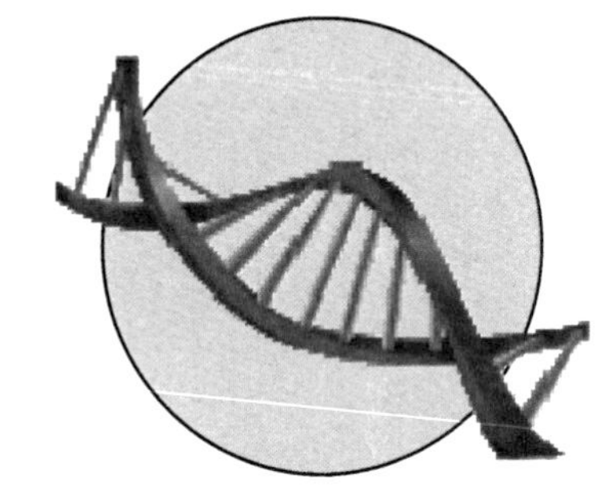

Which aspects of our DNA, our deeper features, are particularly important in managing medical complexity? If we look back at the competencies for the 'Diagnostics' section (see page 60), we see that clinical expertise, problem-solving skills and empathy & sensitivity are important.

There are four major themes in the managing medical complexity domain, each represented by a competence progression, which we will now discuss one by one:

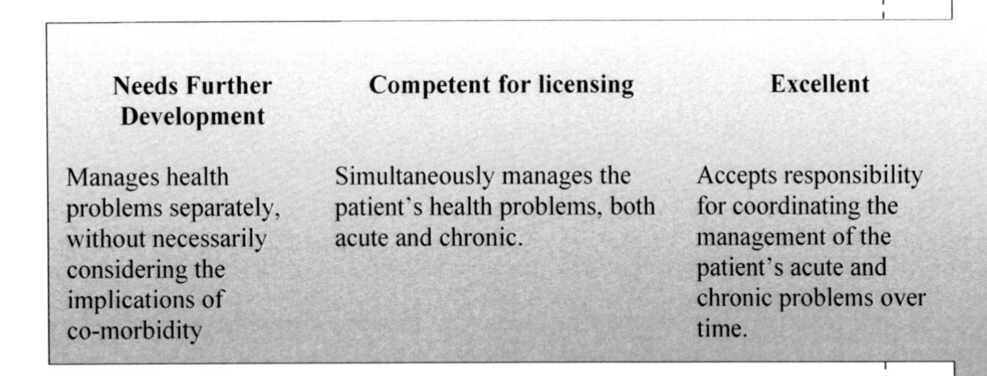

The first progression is principally about learning to deal with simultaneous problems and in particular, dealing with an acute problem against the background of other conditions. We move from:

Managing problems in isolation of each other without considering the potential effects of one problem on another.

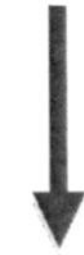

Managing new and existing problems together.

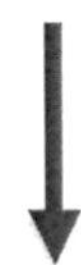

Taking responsibility for orchestrating ongoing management and ensuring that the infrastructure for managing acute and chronic problems in the longer term is adequate.

Looking at each of the word pictures in turn:

Manages health problems separately, without necessarily considering the implications of co-morbidity

Doctors who perform at this basic level tend to be able to identify the patient's problem, but not to look beyond it when they come to develop the management plan. This competency overlaps with holistic care, in which good GPs explore the impact of the patient's problem and try to understand physical, psychological and social aspects before discussing management with the patient. On top of this, in 'managing complexity', we try to gauge how the problem impacts upon other *ongoing* problems and how ongoing problems might have a bearing on the *current* problem or problems. This is what is meant by understanding the 'implications of co-morbidity'.

As we can see, whereas the holistic dimension is patient-orientated and therefore dependent upon the ability to communicate with people, co-morbidity adds a dimension that is dependent on our clinical expertise.

The term 'co-morbidity' sounds like a complicated concept, but it's not and is often recognised independently by patients. For example, when we prescribe for an acute condition it is quite common for patients to ask, 'Will these be okay with my other drugs?' However, patients find it difficult particularly when they are ill, to differentiate between the impact of different *conditions* on their health. Teasing these effects apart is therefore not just a technical skill, but a challenge to our communication skills in helping the patient to understand what we are asking and why.

Tip: How to deal with patients who come with multiple problems

Patients who come with a list are a fact of life! However, we should avoid an inflexible approach such as routinely insisting upon a maximum number of problems per consultation. There may be better ways of managing the situation.

Patients will often test out their GPs before disclosing their hidden agenda/major problem. It's best not to try to deal with *everything*, as this can be exhausting , will make you run late and get stressed. One method is to get the patient to briefly outline the problems at the start of the consultation at which point it may become apparent whether the problems might be linked and which of these might be more urgent (or more serious) than others.

The patient's impression of what's urgent may not be the same as our own and good negotiation skills are required!

Tip: learning to manage co-morbidity

Don't forget to think about the past medical history. It pays dividends to spend a couple of minutes before the patient comes in just to look at: the *list of significant problems* (particularly those coded as being active), the last two or three *consultations* and the *medication* the patient is taking.

An acute illness may be an exacerbation of a chronic disease. Therefore, patients with chronic disease are more likely to have acute illnesses than those patients without this background medical history.

However, acute illness is not always an exacerbation although it is easy to make that assumption. For example, epigastric pain in a patient with peptic ulcer may be a manifestation of ischaemic heart disease. Of equal concern are the situations where the chronic disease can mask the *evolution* of a serious problem. For example, the early signs of bronchogenic carcinoma may be misdiagnosed as exacerbations of COPD. Chronic disease may also influence the *presentation*. Immunocompromised patients may have more severe local & systemic symptoms than might otherwise be expected.

Co-morbidities are often co-chronic, for example diabetics may also be hypertensive. Such patients are subject to polypharmacy and part of management is to streamline the medication to keep it as simple as possible and encourage concordance. Remember that co-morbidity is more common in the elderly, the deprived and in some ethnic groups.

Simultaneously manages the patient's health problems, both acute and chronic.

At this level of performance, we are able to manage co-morbidity *and* are also able to manage more than one problem in the consultation. Even more significantly, we understand the importance of thinking beyond the acute problem by checking for the presence of chronic disease both in the records and by asking the patient. Here are some examples of the impact of an acute condition on the chronic.

Effect on a chronic condition when an acute condition occurs or is treated	Example
Chronic disease medication can't be absorbed	Diarrhoea or vomiting may prevent absorption. Drug interaction between acute and chronic drugs may interfere with absorption
Action of chronic medication interfered with	Chronic medication may become less or more active, for example theophylline levels are decreased by carbamazepine.
Side-effects of chronic treatment are precipitated	In a teenager taking erythromycin for acne, an antihistamine given for hayfever may precipitate arrhythmias.
Chronic condition temporarily becomes worse	For example, a diabetic with cellulitis of the leg might be expected to suffer a temporary deterioration in diabetic control because of the infection. This might even make the patient symptomatic from the diabetes.

Coping with multiple problems simultaneously requires us to identify the other problems going on, usually from the records, and discuss priorities with the patient. The *impact* of one problem upon another, the *risk* this creates along with the patient's *agenda* usually dictate what needs to be done first.

The examples given here have been to do with *physical* illness, but the same principles apply when *mental* health is involved. Most mental health problems are made temporarily worse by intercurrent physical illness and this can be anticipated and managed accordingly. For example, a patient with postnatal depression who was stable on medication before contracting flu, may need to be reviewed sooner than planned to check for deterioration in her mental state.

Accepts responsibility for co-ordinating the management of the patient's acute and chronic problems over time.

This competency falls within the 'excellent' category because 'accepting responsibility' may extend beyond the individual patient and include reviewing/improving the *systems* in the practice that support acute and chronic problem management. This might include the establishment of clinics for chronic diseases and possibly (with Nurse practitioners) for acute conditions. It might also include a review of the communication links so that:

- An adequate summary of the patient's conditions is available at all times including on visits
- An adequate shared patient record is kept and
- Key personnel such as the patient's usual doctor are routinely informed of significant developments.

This competency overlaps with providing continuity of care in that we accept longer-term responsibility, for example by making arrangements to follow through the patient's problem or manage significant problems that may be long-term. The latter requires us to demonstrate our *organisational skills* such as keeping colleagues informed and updating the practice administration systems so that the line of responsibility is clear.

Tip: managing chronic disease

Most major chronic diseases are protocolised, with many being devolved to nurse-run clinics. It is worth finding out how chronic care is organized within the practice. Here are some questions to answer:

- How are patients identified? How are they referred to the clinic?
- What happens within the clinic both with respect to the chronic disease and with other chronic complaints from which the patient suffers?
- Are these dealt with together or separately?
- How is the 'usual doctor' kept informed of the patient's progress?
- What happens if an acute problem is picked up in clinic: to whom is it referred?

Understanding the mechanism of chronic disease management will help you to determine your role in both looking after chronic diseases and in dealing with acute intercurrent problems.

Needs Further Development	Competent for licensing	Excellent	
Draws conclusions when it is appropriate to do so.	Is able to tolerate uncertainty, including that experienced by the patient, where this is unavoidable.	Anticipates and uses strategies for managing uncertainty.	**2**

The second progression concerns how we manage the uncertainty that is an inevitable part of decision-making in primary care. In this, we move from:

Not jumping to conclusions when trying to identify the major problem(s), priorities or possible actions, but exploring the likelihoods until there is sufficient information to give advice or make decisions.

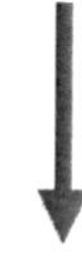

Being able to accept the fact that despite striving to obtain sufficient information, we may still be left with areas of uncertainty and will have to make a judgement on the 'blanks' and act on the basis of what is *probable* rather than what is definite.

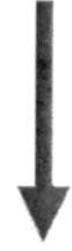

Being able to predict when definite answers or clear guidance are unlikely to be forthcoming and take steps to reduce the adverse effects that this might have on the management plan, the patient and ourselves.

Looking at each of the word pictures in turn:

Draws conclusions when it is appropriate to do so.

In primary care, problem-solving is challenging because patients present with unselected problems that have usually not had the benefit of a doctor's opinion or investigations and may still be in the process of evolving. This is very different from secondary care. It is often not possible, therefore, to exclude a serious condition at the initial consultation and this creates anxiety for both patient and doctor.

Patients and colleagues understand this, which should reduce the anxiety because the emphasis is less on being certain and more on evaluating the probability of what the diagnosis might be, trying to exclude the most dangerous possibilities and developing reasonable management plans with adequate safety nets.

Doctors who act in this way are much less likely to cause avoidable harm. Interestingly, they are also less likely to generate complaints because rather than pull a correct diagnosis like a rabbit from a hat, they talk about the probabilities with their patients as a result of which, they are perceived as being thorough and careful.

How long should we wait before drawing conclusions? In the process of problem solving, we first need to identify the problem(s) and then establish the priorities for action. To identify a problem, we need to allow time for a recognizable pattern to emerge. How long this takes depends upon our:

- Skill in collecting information from history taking, examination and investigation and on our
- Mental library of patterns against which the emerging information can be mapped.

There are obvious dangers with jumping to conclusions. For example, a patient may be wrongly diagnosed with hypertension after one or two moderately-raised blood pressure readings and this could result in the adverse consequences of labelling, treatment and surveillance. However, the converse is also true and it may be risky to wait before taking action even though the information available is scanty. An example of this is when we act on the basis of red flag symptoms or signs, whereby a single symptom such as an isolated postmenopausal vaginal bleed may be enough to trigger referral.

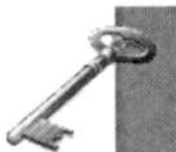

Is able to tolerate uncertainty, including that experienced by the patient, where this is unavoidable.

This competency is thought by educators to be particularly significant in this domain.

Building from the previous competency, in which we demonstrated our ability to judge when to wait and when to act, this competency looks at our ability to cope with the pressure that uncertainty puts upon us. Doctors may be 'coping with uncertainty' simply by being blasé about it. This is why the competency refers to uncertainty that is 'unavoidable', because blasé doctors might inappropriately tolerate uncertainty in situations where the uncertainty is *avoidable* and should be acted upon.

There are a number of ways in which to show that we are coping appropriately. In addition to the ones shown in the box, we should show that our follow-up arrangements and safety-nets are sound and are understood by those involved, in particular the patient.

Anticipates and uses strategies for managing uncertainty.

There are two facets of this competency that mark it out as being more evolved than the previous one. Firstly, whereas the 'competent' descriptor spoke of being able to 'tolerate' uncertainty, at the higher level we have to do more than tolerate or live with it. We now *anticipate* when uncertainty might occur and take action to prevent, reduce or cope with it. Additionally, we need to have a number of ways of dealing with the uncertainty.

Question: when trying to recognize a pattern, why can't we always depend upon the evidence?

The *threshold* for making a diagnosis is often not clear-cut. For example, when does a painful toe with a normal serum uric acid become probable gout?

The *patients* used in research are often not representative of patients in the community. For example, many studies on depression excluded patients who were taking other drugs, had other chronic health problems or drank alcohol. How many depressives do you deal with who fall into this category? It is therefore difficult to extrapolate research findings from an unrepresentative population to our own practice communities.

The *treatments* used in research are often binary because this suits trial designs like RCTs, whereas treatment strategies in primary care are usually multifactorial. For example, children treated for otitis media may receive a combination of parental advice, antipyretic and antibiotic. However, much of the research only considers the antibiotic element.

Question: How might you respond to uncertainty?

Uncertainties should be tolerated in proportion to the evaluation of risk. Our judgment may not be sound if we are overconfident. Keep a check on whether you are overconfident by reflecting on feedback from colleagues and through your portfolio of assessments.

Assessing risk means knowing the red flags (specific symptoms & signs that indicate further action is required) for example in back pain, dyspepsia and headache.

A reflective diary recording consultations where you feel a high degree of uncertainty will help you see where your DENs (doctors educational needs) lie.

We also have to live with the *patient's* uncertainty. For example, the patient may want an x-ray for reassurance, but if it is not clinically indicated we have to resist the temptation to reduce anxiety by investigating more than the situation warrants. Clearly, communication skills are vital if the patient is also to be helped to live with the uncertainty caused by not having (unnecessary) tests.

When might uncertainty be anticipated? The forum of uncertainty is the consultation and we might begin by establishing the patient's health beliefs and in particular, their concerns. In addition to the patient's concerns, we will have concerns of our own and these collective concerns will define the areas in which uncertainty will be particularly difficult to tolerate for one or other party. Having an early discussion about how likely it is that peace of mind will be achieved, which itself might depend upon the diagnostic ability of the tests, will help to prevent expectations becoming inappropriate. For example, a patient presenting with hesitancy of micturition may be worried about prostatic cancer. Discussing what can be achieved from GP tests including PSA would help the doctor and patient decide whether to go for these tests alone or whether referral is likely to be needed irrespective of the tests.

We are in a good position to influence patient expectation, because of our knowledge of probabilities. Therefore, we might anticipate and prevent problems by talking through the natural history of the condition or the way in which it might evolve. This also educates patients about *deviations* from the expected path that should be brought to our attention.

Reducing uncertainty is not done at a single point in time, but is a continuous process that involves data-gathering from tests, guidelines and *discussions* with patients and colleagues in primary and secondary care. Conversing is also a highly effective way of keeping the anxiety caused by uncertainty under control in both patients and doctors.

In the longer term, uncertainty diminishes through experience as we internalise more scripts of how problems evolve and how the significant deviations from what appears 'benign' come to light (e.g. how does dizziness start to look like an acoustic neuroma?; how does anxiety start to look like OCD?)

This might make us think strategically, so that we share these experiences with our colleagues and use the educational process to learn to appropriately manage uncertainty.

Needs Further Development	Competent for Licensing	Excellent	
Appropriately prioritises management approaches, based on an assessment of patient risk.	Communicates risk effectively to patients and involves them in its management to the appropriate degree.	Uses strategies such as monitoring, outcomes assessment and feedback to minimise the adverse effects of risk.	**3**

The third progression deals with patient safety, specifically with how well we gauge risk and how effectively this is shared with the patient. Note that evaluating risk is part of dealing with uncertainty. We move from:

Making an evaluation of risk and on the basis of this, deciding upon appropriate priorities.

Explaining the risk in terms that the patient can understand and to a degree that they can manage, so that the patient can make informed choices where appropriate.

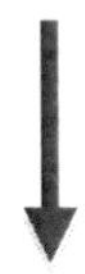

Making plans and using mechanisms to keep patient harm to a minimum.

Looking at each of the word pictures in turn:

Appropriately prioritises management approaches, based on an assessment of patient risk.

We mentioned earlier in this chapter (page 102) how doctors can decide with the patient which problems to prioritise. The next stage of dialogue is to formulate management approaches that seem reasonable from a medical point of view.

Patients can't help with this aspect of risk analysis because either they do not have medical expertise, or if they do, they can't be objective about themselves. However, they can help by being open about their symptoms so that risk can be adequately gauged, rather than playing the symptoms down, e.g. to avoid admission to hospital.

The management approaches that are then discussed with the patient should, first and foremost, be the safest available given the known facts.

Assessing patient risk isn't simply a matter of establishing the medical diagnosis. Patients may also be at risk for social reasons e.g. if they are depressed and can't self-manage or be adequately supervised. Therefore, whereas an elderly patient with bronchopneumonia who was living with her daughter could be treated at home, a widow with only elderly neighbours for support might require domiciliary nursing or hospital admission.

Risk assessment also comes into play when deciding on the pros and cons of treatment. For instance, a decision on the drug management of depression (nowadays, a contentious issue) might be influenced by an objective depression score. Formal risk assessment is becoming a more prominent feature of chronic disease management as a method of gauging the overall impact of many factors on disease progression. Chronic heart and chronic kidney disease are conditions where multifactorial analysis converts risk to a percentage and a category respectively. These analyses can then guide how intensively the patient's condition needs to be managed and therefore how much of a medical priority the problem becomes.

Communicates risk effectively to patients and involves them in its management to the appropriate degree.

As we progress, the challenge is to explain the risk factors, put them in proportion with each other and importantly, prevent misunderstanding. For example we may

Tip: example of risk assessment from the curriculum on sexual health

- Use the sexual history (including partner history and information on sexual practices including condom use) and other relevant information to assess risk of sexually transmitted infection, unwanted pregnancy and cervical cancer.
- Use risk assessment to tailor advice and care accordingly, including advice on safer sexual practices and Hepatitis B immunisation.
- Be aware of factors which may indicate that a woman is at high risk of cervical cancer and the value of an opportunistic approach to screening in this group.

need to explain to patients with CKD3 that they are not suffering from kidney failure and in need of dialysis or a renal transplant! Checking what the patient has understood may seem unnecessary, particularly when they have been smiling and nodding during the explanation, but as this example shows, it is vital when risk is being explained.

Once we have explained the data on risk, we next need to discuss the *implications* such as the pros and cons of different legitimate approaches and do so in a way that allows patients to take part in the management decision to the *appropriate degree*. This last phrase is important because in some situations (for example, emergency admission for chest pain) our aim may be simply to inform the patient of what needs to be done and why, rather than get them to make a choice where, actually, no legitimate choice exists.

Good communication skills are important, because risk causes *fear*. Language is important, so for example we might talk about 'the *chances* of' rather than 'the *risk* of'. Again, establishing the patient's concerns will help us to guide the explanation appropriately so that these concerns can be addressed and wherever possible, minimized.

Often, the explanation of risk will cover what might happen (particularly, what might go wrong) in different situations including what might happen if *nothing* was done. We might also discuss the possible timescale. Sometimes, the explanation may require a diagram or picture and occasionally the use of numbers and percentages. If we remember to ask, patients can usually guide us about which approach they prefer. Studies have shown that numbers are often better understood when presented in pictorial form, such as two sad faces and 98 smiley faces, representing a 2% risk of a particular adverse outcome. People also understand medical risk better when it is compared to something they have an intuitive feeling about, such as 'the chances of being struck by lightning'. If needed, the discussion can be supported by patient information materials such as leaflets and websites.

Not infrequently when a genuine choice is being offered, patients will ask for our opinion as to what they should do. If we're sure that they are not asking this because they haven't understood our explanation, then one way forward is to say what we would choose for *ourselves*, making it clear that this is not a recommendation of what the patient should do.

Assessor's corner: does the doctor try to learn from the outcomes of risk management?

The outcomes may be gauged *indirectly* from audit, case review and feedback from those involved in the patient's care and *directly* from the patient and patient's family.

If the doctor claims to have learned from the management of risk, which methods has s/he used? Which were the most helpful and why? Does the doctor try to pass these valuable lessons on to others? How?

Uses strategies such as monitoring, outcomes assessment and feedback to minimise the adverse effects of risk.

In practice, much of risk reduction depends upon the quality of our follow-up arrangements and safety-netting. As ever, good communication and record keeping are important so that both patient and clinicians are aware of the degree of risk, the timescale for improvement and the circumstances under which the patient should be reviewed.

When the risk is more complicated or potentially more serious, the management approach may need to be explained to the patient more detail, with supporting information and possibly with another family member or carer sitting in attendance. For example, think about how you would explain risk to an asthmatic with cardiac failure who is being initiated on a beta-blocker.

'Outcomes assessment' means learning from the outcome of a particular management approach by weighing up the positive and negative outcomes. In general practice, the outcomes may not be simply the physical or psychological benefits or the adverse effects. Because we are interested in the *impact* of illness, the outcomes may include the holistic elements of the effects on everyday life, work, schooling and social relationships.

Learning from these measures might help the patient's future care to be tailored appropriately and would also help us to improve treatment for *other* patients with similar problems.

Needs Further Development	Competent for licensing	Excellent
Maintains a positive attitude to the patient's health.	Consistently encourages improvement and rehabilitation and, where appropriate, recovery. Encourages the patient to participate in appropriate health promotion and disease prevention strategies.	Coordinates a team based approach to health promotion, prevention, cure, care and palliation and rehabilitation.

4

The fourth progression concerns the attitude that we have towards promoting health and the skills we use in doing so. We move from:

Recognizing the difference between treating disease and managing health. Developing a positive approach to promoting health.

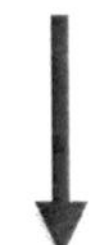

To this positive attitude, adding the skills to motivate the patient and to encourage participation in more formal health promoting activities.

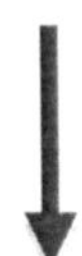

Looking beyond the individual and helping to develop and coordinate a team approach to health promotion as part of a spectrum of care that we offer our community.

Looking at each of the word pictures in turn:

Maintains a positive attitude to the patient's health.

As doctors, we spend the majority of our training recognizing illness and disease (real and imagined). For many specialties, treating disease in order to restore health is the limit of the doctors concern. For GPs the duty is wider because we have a remit to not only restore but also to maintain and improve health within the individual and within our practice communities.

What does this mean in practice? A useful starting point is to consider a definition of health, such as that provided by the World Health Organization (WHO). It states that

'Health is a state of complete physical, mental and social well-being and not merely the absence of disease or infirmity'.

This is worth remembering. In more recent years, this statement has been modified to include the ability to lead a *'socially and economically productive life'*. The WHO definition is not without criticism, as some argue that health cannot be defined as a *state* at all, but must be seen as a *process* of continuous adjustment to the changing demands of living and of the changing meanings we give to life. The WHO definition is therefore considered by many as an idealistic goal rather than a realistic proposition.

Question: What are the factors that influence your attitude to the patient's health?

Your understanding of what health means.

Your personal experience of health and expectations for your own future health.

Your attitudes, behaviour and experience regarding the maintenance of your own physical and mental health, (diet, exercise, hygiene, stress management and disease prevention).

Your expectations of health in the practice population based on personal experience and on the expectations of others, including government, employers, profession, colleagues and society.

Your expectations of health in a particular individual, based on previous experiences with the patient.

The patient's attitudes, behaviour and capacity to change.

The resources available to meet any proposed plan.

The WHO definition also speaks in absolutes. We could argue that no one is ever in a state of 'complete....... well-being' and in real life, most people describe themselves in relative terms, e.g. as being healthy when they are mostly, rather than completely in this state, or healthy when compared to how they have been or how other people are.

Interestingly, many people adjust to their infirmities and may regard themselves as being healthy when their background conditions are in a state of control and not significantly impairing function Thus, patients with mild osteoarthritis who are controlled on simple analgesia may regard themselves as being healthy. Provided that this does not result in clinicians becoming complacent by taking the patient's view at face value, this mindset can be very helpful.

The worry is that patients, sometimes through ignorance, may accept a lower expectation of health than need be the case. Part of our role is to challenge these expectations. For example, patients may accept their symptoms of heartburn and may simply use over-the-counter antacids when required even though these are not the most effective treatments. A PPI prescription from the GP may transform their expectation of health by effectively curing them of their symptoms.

This competency is about our attitude to the patient's health and there are a number of factors that will influence this (see box on the left). Look through the factors and think of examples from your own personal and working lives. In particular, think about your personal biases i.e. your likes, dislikes and prejudices. Next, think about what it is about you that helps you to have a positive attitude to health (your *helpers*) and which factors get in the way (your *hinderers*). You may need to work on both by increasing the use you make of the former and thinking of ways to get rid of or reduce the impact of the latter. Once you have a better understanding of *yourself*, you are more likely to develop an approach that will help your patients.

It goes without saying that having a positive approach to health is a 'good thing', but it is worth asking *why* our attitude to health is so important. Patients are not only given treatment by doctors but, particularly in general practice, are powerfully influenced by our attitudes and expectations. If patients have a positive approach to their own health, they are more likely to cope psychologically and partly as a result of this, restore function more quickly. There is widespread anecdotal evidence that physical recovery may also be enhanced. So how do we develop an approach that helps our patients?

Let's firstly consider the context. Particularly in western society, there is widespread anxiety about disease, which in objective terms can seem disproportionate to the reality. Because of medical technology, there are high expectations that doctors will cure rather than palliate and that technology will provide a 'pill for every ill'. Coupled with this, people feel less in control of their own lives and thereby less able to cope by using their own resources.

Of course, this is a generalisation but when we think about the patient's health, we often do so against this background. To help the patient, we need to understand their attitudes to health and self-care and their expectations of us. When these are understood, we are in a better position to educate and empower, where these are appropriate.

In particular, the patient can be encouraged to have greater confidence in their own powers of recuperation and there may be a need here for education as well as advice. Patients may need help with understanding what we mean by a healthy lifestyle.

More broadly we have an important role, particularly in secular society, of helping the patient to see health in psychological, social and spiritual dimensions as well as in the physical one. To give a practical example, one of the main determinants of health for any human being is the feeling that we are valued by others around us. Being valued can vary from being a mother, earning money, helping to redecorate a relative's flat, to providing advice and so on.

No matter what the objective level of health, it is nearly always possible for people to make a contribution of some value to those around them. Although it sounds bizarre, this can include the time before death, where the way in which patients conduct themselves in facing their final illness can provide a powerful legacy to the next generation. GPs can share such thoughts and bring hope and motivation in situations where these are not immediately apparent. Often, this can do as much to relieve suffering as more conventional treatments.

This competency speaks of doctors *maintaining* a positive attitude. This is because there are times in looking after the patient when it can be hard to be positive. For example, the patient's demeanour and attitude may be off-putting, the mood may be depressed, the illness may be serious and the outlook bleak. Additionally, we may lack motivation or interest. Each of these will demand attention so that the patient can be supported in developing an attitude that helps them cope better. Remember that there is *always* something we can offer (see page 30).

Consistently encourages improvement and rehabilitation and, where appropriate, recovery.

This competency builds on the preceding one by adding the knowledge and skills to encourage patients to improve.

Some of these skills have been touched upon above and include the ability to reflect on our attitudes and to get patients to think about their own ideas and expectations regarding health. For example, when problems become chronic, patients can lose heart or genuinely believe that recovery is not possible. Through education and motivation, we can help the patient to challenge this view and turn themselves around. For example, a patient who is breathless on exertion and suffering mild hip pain may feel that 'living with it' is the only option. However, it may be that weight reduction and regular manageable exercise would both improve cardio-respiratory fitness and reduce the load on the hips, thereby helping both conditions to improve.

We have to encourage patients without lying to them and as we see from the wording of the competency, recovery or cure will not always be possible. In these situations, we may encourage the patient by describing what improvement means in terms of the benefits to their everyday lives. Therefore, in encouraging diabetic patients about diet and exercise, they may be less impressed (although pleased) with good blood sugar and blood pressure readings than with feeling more energetic when their condition is better controlled.

What we learn from this is that whilst objective measures matter to doctors, they may be less motivating for patients than their subjective improvements. It is therefore worth asking patients who are improving from some condition, to

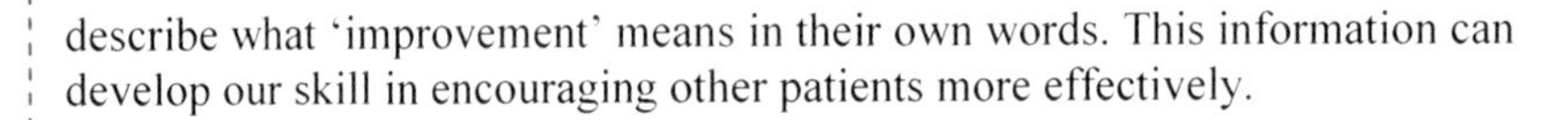

describe what 'improvement' means in their own words. This information can develop our skill in encouraging other patients more effectively.

Encourages the patient to participate in appropriate health promotion and disease prevention strategies.

Like the previous one, this competency is also in the 'competent' column. Doctors who perform at this level know which health promotion and disease prevention strategies are recommended and are available locally. Often, practical knowledge of how to access these services is also needed so that patients know, for example, how to get one-to-one smoking cessation advice in the locality.

We also need to know about other strategies at local or national level. For example, the curriculum identifies screening strategies in women's health including those for cervical, breast and ovarian cancer. Screening programmes also apply to postnatal depression and osteoporosis.

Coordinates a team-based approach to health promotion, prevention, cure, care and palliation and rehabilitation.

This competency is categorised as 'excellent' because we have moved beyond thinking about what we personally can do for the patient. We have also moved beyond thinking about the *individual* patient. At this level, we now think about how health promotion fits with other parts of the spectrum of care and how it is addressed by various members of the team, rather than by doctors alone. In other words, we think about the *system* of care and how this can be developed and coordinated to help the practice community.

Learning about the spectrum of care from the curriculum

By 'spectrum of care', we mean the following range: prevention....health promotion....curing patients....providing care....rehabilitation....palliation

Irrespective of whether patients can be cured, there is always something within this spectrum that can be offered. The spectrum could be thought of as a patient pathway or journey. The curriculum suggests that we:

'Describe the risks to patient safety by considering an illness pathway/journey in which a variety of healthcare professionals have been involved. In particular, reflect on the interface issues arising from the current multitude of such providers and be able to comment on the ways in which, as a GP, you can work to minimise these'

In primary care, chronic diseases provide good examples of a team-based approach from which we can learn. Using diabetes as an example, we can learn about how the connections are made between

- Disease prevention (e.g. through the management of obesity by dieticians or foot care by chiropodists)
- Health promotion (smoking cessation from pharmacists)
- Providing diabetic care (e.g. diabetic nurse specialists) and
- Palliation (district nurses).

Each of these facets of the spectrum (prevention, cure etc) may be witnessed in secondary care training as well as in primary care. Look out for examples when you are working in hospital. Some posts are more obviously geared up, for example time spent in medicine of the elderly will provide opportunities to witness care, palliation & rehabilitation. This may help you to identify the gaps that you need to address in other hospital training posts and in primary care.

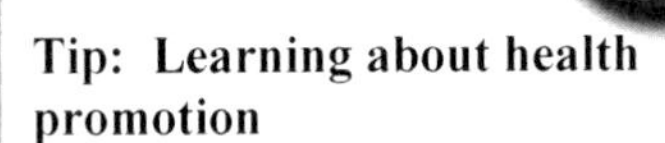

Tip: Learning about health promotion

You need to get local knowledge and find out what is available, because once you have this you can convert a positive attitude into practical suggestions.

Many practices have health promotion/disease prevention activities available, often in special clinics. Find out what these are and how they are accessed.

These might include immunisation, travel clinics, sexual health screening and family-planning clinics. Health promotion also takes place as a routine part of other clinics, for example diet, exercise and lifestyle advice is given in new patient clinics. Clinicians are also prompted with certain health checks (e.g. smoking cessation) through computer prompts, especially when linked to the quality outcome framework (QOF).

Are there other health promotion activities that you feel should be undertaken? Why? How could this be done? Before answering this, look for any special characteristics in your practice population that might suggest particular health risks.

To learn about teamwork, look out for examples in practice, evaluate others doing it and talk to the practice manager. Also, try it out by being a team leader on a practice project and remember to ask for constructive feedback on your performance!

Our role is to:

- Recognize and understand the various elements of the spectrum
- Review who is best placed to attend to each element
- Encourage a coordinated approach by building an infrastructure, providing training and the necessary resources and finally
- Review the effectiveness of the system through audit and feedback.

This sounds a mighty task, but it's the way in which you can translate what you have learned from the other competencies in this progression to a much larger practice population, thus benefiting your whole community.

You'll find that many of the 'excellent' descriptors in the competencies framework are designed to help you to take what you have learned from individual patient care and apply it to populations, maximising the positive impact of your abilities.

Assessor's corner

To demonstrate this competency, the doctor should be seen as being *proactive*.

The doctor should raise the patient's longer term health as an issue in the consultation, motivating the patient to have a positive attitude to health and to take action to preserve it.

Look at how the doctor behaves on COT. Is health promotion on the doctor's radar?

Does the doctor have positive approach to recovery etc, perhaps with verbal and non-verbal evidence of encouragement?

Does the doctor have any practical suggestions?

Do these show knowledge of resources in the practice and the locality?

Management

11 Management: Overview of the performance areas

Management is the third of the RDMp clusters and is made up of three domains from the competence framework, these being:

- Primary care administration and IMT
- Community orientation
- Maintaining performance, learning and teaching

The term management is used here in a broad sense and as Tim Norfolk points out it is related to the wider handling of our professional responsibilities to patients and colleagues, i.e. it is not simply related to the administrative work that our practice managers undertake. (Norfolk TD, Siriwardena AN. A unifying theory of general practice: relationship, diagnostics, management and professionalism (RDM-p) *Quality in Primary Care* 2009; **17**)

To understand our management skills, let's think of them as the filling in the following sandwich. Firstly, we must accept that the broad area of management is part of our personal responsibility as doctors. By accepting this responsibility, we are demonstrating an important aspect of professionalism, which we discuss in more detail in the section on 'Fitness to practise' on page 199. This is the top layer of the sandwich.

Next come the management skills, which comprise the filling. In more detail:

Management is all about improving outcomes by exercising the right amount of influence or control. It refers to our ability to manage issues, events, relationships and ourselves over time.

The first requirement is learning which situations are readily amenable to being managed and which are less easily influenced. The spectrum is broad, for example we might *manage episodes* such as the sequence of events in a consultation or *ongoing situations* such as our responsibilities as the leader of a project. We can also use management skills with *relationships*, for example by planning to develop a relationship of trust with the patient through continuity of care, or with colleagues through discussion on how to work together effectively. Importantly, management skills include the ability to continually keep track of situations and adjust to them. For example, we 'manage' ourselves by *monitoring* our performance and professional development and more widely, by monitoring our mental and physical well-being.

By so doing, we take steps to work as effectively as we can and keep doing so throughout our careers. To be effective at management, we also need to learn that our influence has a narrow therapeutic range. Too little brings no benefit whereas too much can be toxic to ourselves and the people around us!

The final layer of the sandwich is the realisation that we and the situations we are involved with, such as the treatment of patients, are influenced by *other* people's attempts to manage. Just as we try to exercise some control in order to improve the outcomes, others around us do the same and part of our professionalism is to fit in with this to the appropriate degree. To give a clinical example, a colleague may suggest to the patient that if the symptoms did not improve, certain tests or a referral may be needed. We would certainly need to consider these thoughts and maybe 'fit in' with the colleague's plan.

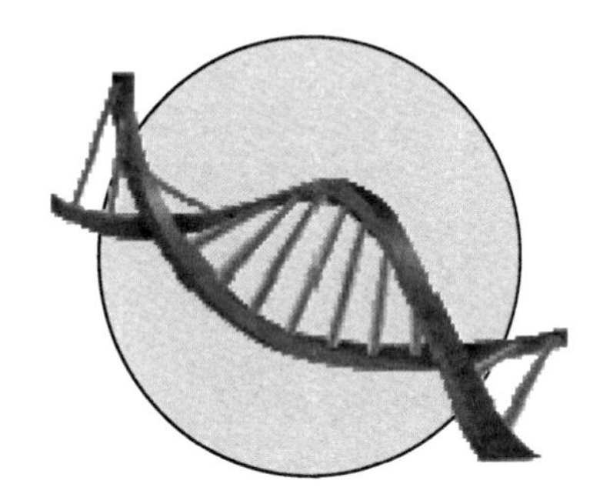

The deeper features are our DNA. Although few in number, they underpin all the behaviours described in the competence framework and are described in terms of knowledge, skills, attitudes and personal qualities. The behaviours being tested in the 'Management section are shown in the table below, where the categories indicate the degree of weighting.

The behaviours are shown in the left-hand column. We will describe these in greater detail to clarify what they are. As you read them, use the table to cross-reference them to the domains that they underpin. This will increase your understanding and help you to develop the skills you need for each area of performance. The weighting will help you here. For example 'community orientation' requires problem-solving skills and the ability to cope with pressure (e.g. from the conflict created by rationing decisions) whereas primary-care administration and IMT do not.

If you are (or your trainee is) having a problem with performance in a domain, look at the deeper features for guidance on where the problem might lie and therefore which behaviours need working on.

	Primary care administration and IMT	Community orientation	Maintaining performance, learning and teaching
Clinical expertise			Low
Problem-solving skills		Medium	Low
Empathy & sensitivity	Low		
Team involvement & managing others		Low	Medium
Learning & personal development			High
Coping with pressure		Low	
Organisation & planning	Medium		

Clinical expertise

Uses evidence from guidelines, medical literature and audit activity to inform clinical judgement.

Problem-solving skills

Trying not to have a restricted mindset, but *thinking around issues.* For example, in trying to understand the epidemiological, social, economic and ethnic features of the local population and what effect (positive and negative) these features might have on healthcare.

From a mass of detailed and complex information, being able to *identify key points*, for example the most relevant features of the local community that might have an impact on the doctor's services. Similarly, identifying the key points from research and guidelines that are relevant and transposable to the care of our local population.

Being *open to new ideas/possibilities.* For instance, rather than just accepting that healthcare is the way it is, being prepared to think about changes both in terms of what is needed and what is possible and being able to suggest changes, for example by describing new forms of service delivery in the community. Likewise, being open to new ideas on patient management as suggested by the medical literature

In situations of complexity such as the dilemmas created by rationing ,trying to square the needs of individual patients with the needs of the community, being able to *use an ethical framework* to problem-solve. Also, given a mass of information from guidelines, research and audit, being able to use a framework to decide what the data shows and what weight it carries. These are the problem-solving skills of *critical appraisal.*

Empathy & sensitivity

Having a co-operative and inclusive approach, for instance in taking care to make records that others find useful.

Showing sensitivity to the patient by making efforts to counter the adverse effects on communication and relationship of using the computer in consultation.

Team involvement & managing others

Being *participative, non-confrontational and flexible*, for instance when dealing with rationing or talking about commissioning within a group of local providers. Similarly, *working collaboratively* with colleagues to learn from audit and significant events.

Negotiating and *being consistent* so that decisions are not unfairly influenced by prejudice or the pressure generated by those who can lobby most effectively.

With clinical governance, respecting the views of others, being prepared to *compromise* in order to achieve improvements.

Delegating and showing leadership where these are appropriate.

Learning and personal development

Being able to learn from experience, using this to *acknowledge limitations and identify learning needs.*

Continually *monitoring* performance.

Keeping *regularly updated* on clinical and other job-related skills in line with the changing GP role

Coping with pressure

Remaining *calm and under control* in situations of tension for example when, in the face of anger or opposition, deciding how limited resources should be used . Similarly, when faced with the demands of patients for time, attention and resources that the doctor may not feel are reasonable.

Not losing sight of the wider needs of situation, for example in balancing the needs of individual patients with the health needs of the local community.

Organisation & planning:

The ability to understand what the administration & computing systems are capable of doing and *working within these capacities.*

Organize information in a structured and planned manner, for example with medical record-keeping.

Recognize deficiencies and limitations in the IT and admin systems and *recommend appropriate changes.*

Being able to think ahead about what might be needed in the future and on the basis of this, make appropriate plans for the populations healthcare needs.

Understanding limitations and constraints, for example *limited healthcare resources*, and being able to work within them.

Understanding where priorities are in conflict with each other and being able to *make appropriate choices,* for example between the needs of the patient and the needs of the wider community.

12 Management: Primary care administration and information management and technology

This competency area is about the appropriate use of primary care administration systems, effective record keeping and information technology for the benefit of patient care.

At first glance, this section might appear rather dull compared to the other performance areas as it doesn't seem to be directly related to patient care. We might even ask 'What has 'primary care administration' to do with me and my training as a doctor?' However, for modern GPs, the protocols and systems on which primary care is based are as essential to the care of patients as sound clinical skills. As doctors, we have a vital role in developing the systems that meet our needs.

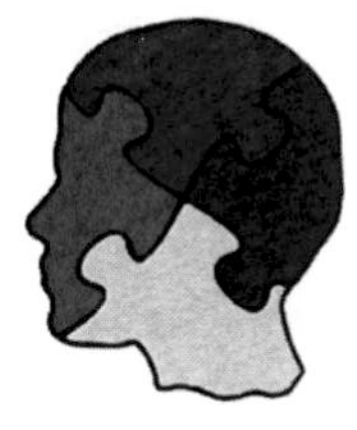

Joined up?
See p14

For licensing, we are not expected to have an in-depth knowledge of practice management, but we should understand the basics of practice administration system and in particular, the role of the GP in applying, monitoring and improving this so that patient care is optimized and the practice, as a business, runs smoothly (and profitably!).

Computing skills on the other hand, are as essential in modern practice as being able to write, and the curriculum requires us to have a level of skill equivalent to the ECDL (European computer driving licence).

This performance area also includes the ability to keep good medical records, which is partly a matter of attitude and partly a skill.

Which aspects of our DNA, our deeper features, are particularly important in Primary care administration and IMT? If we look back at the competencies for the Management section (page 118), we see that organisation & planning and to a lesser degree, empathy & sensitivity are important.

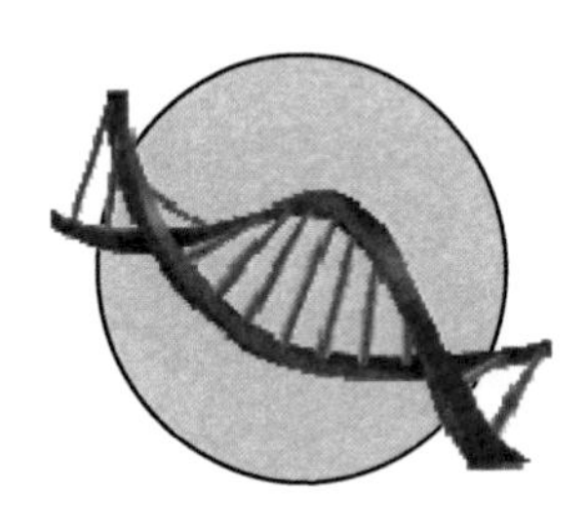

There are three major themes in the Primary care administration and IMT performance area, each represented by a progression, which we will now discuss one by one:

Needs Further Development	Competent for licensing	Excellent
Demonstrates a rudimentary understanding of the organisation of primary care and the use of primary care computer systems.	Uses the primary care organisational and IMT systems routinely and appropriately in patient care.	Uses and modifies organisational and IMT systems to facilitate: • Clinical care to individuals and communities • Clinical governance • Practice administration

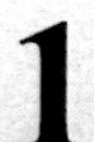

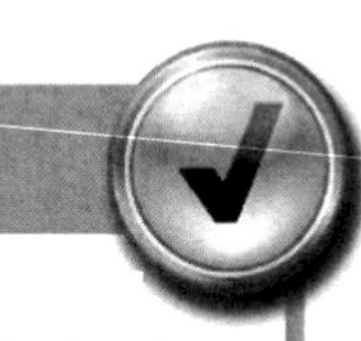

Tip: knowing the legislation

The legislation does not need to be known in depth, but there are some important Acts and protocols that you should be aware of:

The Data protection Act.

Access to medical reports Act
The practice confidentiality policies. In particular, you should find out: who has access to the medical records? what level of data do they have access to? who is allowed to make changes? how these changes verified? (e.g. additions to repeat medication), how is record access audited? what are the sanctions for proven breach of confidentiality?

Freedom of information Act.

The first progression is principally about understanding and using the administrative and computing systems in the practice. We move from:

Having a basic understanding of how the practice is managed and the computing system that the practice uses

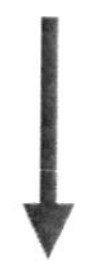

Making use of the practice administration systems and the computer systems on a routine basis and doing so appropriately

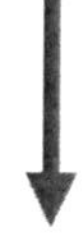

Having a deeper understanding of how clinical care, monitoring systems and practice management are dependent on administration and IT systems. Additionally, using this understanding to suggest improvements.

Looking at each of the competencies in turn:

Demonstrates a rudimentary understanding of the organisation of primary care and the use of primary care computer systems.

As the competency suggests, our level of understanding need not be great but should be sufficient for us to understand the structure of practice management including the roles and responsibilities of those involved, i.e. managers, secretaries, receptionists, IT personnel etc. On the computing side, we should understand the nature of IT in primary care including the uses to which it is put by patients and healthcare professionals and the special provisions made to protect data storage and access.

For example, we should know in general terms about the types of data *collected*, how these are *collated* and used for management and clinical purposes and how the practice IT *connects* with inter and intranets and allows data transfer with authorised agencies such as hospitals and community pharmacies. We also need to understand how computing is changing to allow national accessibility of NHS data through the electronic care record and the opportunities and threats that this brings.

Uses the primary care organisational and IMT systems routinely and appropriately in patient care.

The first competency was about the general principles and making sure we 'understand'. The 'competent' descriptor is concerned with whether we can apply this understanding to practice. The curriculum usefully lays out a number of specific IM&T skills that need to be acquired:

At the end of their general practice training, the GP should be able to:

Demonstrate an ability to use the practice clinical system effectively and routinely for tasks such as prescribing, entering clinical data , processing pathology results, making referrals and accessing data

Comments: When you first joined the practice, you should have had an introduction to the computing system. Whoever does this initial training might also be able to advise you how to monitor your progress with learning to use the system. They may be able to collate feedback regarding e.g. when information is not entered (such as a new repeat prescription) or properly coded (such as a disease or referral) and problems then arise. You should also go through your early consultations with someone who is system-literate to check that you are using the computer appropriately and maximising the things that it can usefully do for you.

Demonstrate awareness of coding systems in current use for effective record keeping

Comment: Coding is the backbone of retrieval and audit. Practices use READ coding and of the many thousands of possible codes, the practice will use a relatively small number of agreed codes, some of which are mandated by external systems such as QOF. As well as *clinical* codes, there will be others that are necessary for *administrative* purposes. For example, a code may be entered when a letter is dictated so that an audit trail is begun. Similarly, for *financial* management a code may be used when an insurance extract or pre-employment medical is undertaken.

Demonstrate the effective use of templates for protocol-delivered activities such as the management of chronic disease, health promotion and risk assessment

Comment: protocols are usually produced in-house either de novo or by adapting a protocol used elsewhere. Practice managers and nurses often share such information between practices but local adaptation is usually needed because practices collate and use their data in different ways. To demonstrate effective use, you should firstly know whether there *is* a protocol that should be used. Usually, you will be prompted by the computer that a protocol is available and asked whether you wish to use it or not. Human nature being what it is, templates do not get filled in if practitioners are not motivated to do so. For trainees, the financial incentive of maximising income through data collection will not be there, but because it is good for patient care and is valued by colleagues, you should still try to attend to computer prompts, such as (in England) the alerts regarding missing QOF data.

To understand the clinical importance of templates, look at the data items that the template requires you to collect and ask yourself *why* these have been chosen. For example, patients with enduring mental illness often have physical illnesses that may be overlooked. This may be because of the dominance of the mental problems, prejudice, difficulty with dealing with them or because health promotion is not actively pursued.

Therefore, the template for the chronic disease management of such patients may ask the expected questions about control of the mental condition, medication review and care plans but may also ask about blood pressure monitoring, screening for ischaemic heart disease, diabetes and so on. Ask yourself what might happen if the templates were not completed. Who loses out and how can this be avoided?

Demonstrate the use of call/recall systems within the practice to the benefit of patient care

Comment: What are the situations in which medical surveillance is necessary? Increasingly, GPs take over the routine surveillance of medical conditions and medications that were once the province of secondary care. For example, chronic kidney disease and insulin dependent diabetes are dealt with in the community. Likewise, drugs such as azathioprine and warfarin can be monitored by the practice sometimes supported by shared-care protocols between primary and secondary care.

Call and recall systems can be used for any situation that requires predictable periodic patient review. A system is especially important where the patient might come to harm if a review is missed for example:

- monitoring thyroid function where biochemical abnormality will occur well before any symptoms or

- bone scanning every few years in patients with osteoporosis, where the follow-up period is long and likely to be forgotten.

Understand the criteria for good data entry including timeliness, appropriateness and accuracy and the connection between this and improved patient health outcomes

Comment: the major purpose of good data entry is to ensure that patient health outcomes are improved. You could both learn what this means *and* demonstrate many of the skills in this performance area by conducting a clinical audit.

Understand the application of the electronic record to analyse data and monitor outcomes, identify trends and warn of deteriorating performance, provide continuous auditing

Provide appropriate prompts to action and reduce risk by warning of potentially adverse outcomes, for example when prescribing. Provide population based call and recall systems, for example in screening

Share information appropriately and securely with the healthcare team

Comment: one of the great advances that data management brings is the opportunity to look at trends and identify problems whilst they are developing and before they become a significant clinical issue. In the past, this could only be done retrospectively e.g. in response to periodic audits or to significant events. One way to look at continuous auditing is to examine, for English practices, QMAS (Quality Management and Analysis System) which can be accessed from the practice computers. This is a national IT system which gives GP practices and Primary Care Trusts objective evidence and feedback on the quality of care delivered to patients. It supports the Quality and Outcomes element of the GP contract and has been in operation since 2004. The system shows practices during the course of each reporting year, how they are progressing in meeting their targets.

How can it be used? An example is that if it is seen that control of blood pressure or blood sugar in diabetics is starting to fall short of the standard, action can be taken to direct attention and resources to the problem.

Demonstrate the use the practice's computer system to improve the quality of care both at the level of the individual and that of the practice

Demonstrate effective use of inter-agency systems such as Pathology links with secondary care, protocol links to the primary care organisations, for example to access local formularies and guidelines, and GP-GP record transfer

Comment: if the practice has not already done so, you could create links to formularies and guidelines perhaps on your computer desktop, through 'favourites' in the Internet browser or by placing links on a shared file that the whole practice can access.

Demonstrate effective use of expert and web-based information systems e.g. MENTOR & PRODIGY

Demonstrate the use of the computer for practice-based searches and audit

Use IM&T in the management of multiple complaints and pathologies, both acute and chronic health problems e.g. by effective use of the medical record and by seeking the best evidence in practice

Comment: you should think about how you use the medical record to improve patient care. Although it is understandable because of the time pressures in each consultation, it is still disappointing that comparatively little use is made of IT to improve decision-making and patient care.

For example, attendances for the same coded problem can be viewed together, thereby illustrating how the problem has evolved. This can uncover important patterns that might otherwise be difficult to see and which the patient may not have pieced together. For example, a patient with occasional chest infections treated by a number of doctors over the preceding two years, may actually have COPD. This becomes a more obvious differential diagnosis when the pattern of consultations is clear.

Information from the patient narrative can also be cross-referenced to the prescribing history. Therefore, it may become quickly apparent that a dry recurrent cough came on shortly after an ACEI was commenced. For patients with multiple pathologies, it is now very much quicker with computers to scan the past medical history and to appreciate which problems are currently active. This need only take a few seconds before the patient comes into the room and can quickly place the patient's problem within the background context, thus helping us to stop dealing with each attendance as a separate and unrelated event when actually, it is part of a pattern that is emerging.

Demonstrate the use of IM&T to access community–based resources e.g. voluntary organisations and self-help groups

Use IM&T to share information and coordinate patient care with other health professionals

The 'organisational' skills that need to be acquired relate to knowing and observing the agreed practice routines so as to facilitate the running of the practice. This will extend from knowing who does what and involving team and staff members appropriately, to knowing the areas in which practice protocols exist and following these when required.

The organisational and computing systems are also essential to patient care, risk management and the financial security of the practice and those whose livelihoods depend upon it. As an illustration of these points, because of the link between care and income mediated through data reporting, a failure to code a patient's condition appropriately may result in the need for immunisation not being identified (poor clinical care) and clinical targets not being met (poor financial return).

Uses and modifies organisational and IMT systems to facilitate:

- **Clinical care to individuals and communities**
- **Clinical governance**
- **Practice administration**

The previous competency was heavily concerned with 'using' the systems whereas this, under the excellent column, takes this to another level that requires us to understand the systems well enough to *modify* them in line with perceived need.

Learning from practice meetings (see box below) is a good way of observing the practicalities of organisational change. These meetings also help us to learn where the impetus for such changes comes from. Sometimes, it can be from PCO priorities and opportunities to improve care, at other times from practice business needs and occasionally from the need to reduce risk, perhaps prompted by a significant event.

Making changes

This criterion is important, because without the ability to modify systems, practices cannot improve their services. A good place to learn how this is done is in meetings that involve doctors and managers in which new developments or changing demands are discussed.

If the practice decides that the service needs to be improved, some form of project management then takes place whereby administration protocols and computing systems are produced or modified. Try to attend these meetings, listen out for proposed changes and look closely at the action points.

Try to follow the simpler ones through so that you can learn about the practicalities of making such changes. There are nearly always unforeseen complications and unintended consequences which may mean that the systems need further tweaking.

The categories in the word picture are not mutually exclusive. For example, the medical literature may suggest that carers are relatively unsupported and that through neglect of their own health, they have an increased risk of morbidity that could be avoided. The practice may then decide to keep a carers' register and develop a protocol for capturing carers' details and proactively offer advice on support services and health checks for those who are not already under medical care. In this example, 'clinical care to individuals and communities' is improved.

To give a further example, the PCO might be keen to improve the medical surveillance of nursing homes through an 'enhanced service' contract. The practice may be willing to take on responsibility for a large number of nursing home patients, to draw up care plans and make arrangements for routine medical review. This would be an additional service to that already provided for the practice's patients and would meet a locality need whilst improving practice income.

In this example, the administration and computing changes would have to meet the needs of the new service, but would also have to be capable of generating information that would assure an external body such as the PCO that the service being offered was of a sufficiently high standard.

Needs Further Development	Competent for licensing	Excellent	
Uses the computer record and online information during the consultation.	Uses the computer during the consultation whilst maintaining rapport with the patient.	Incorporates the computer records and online information in the consultation to improve communication with the patient.	**2**

The second progression is about learning to use electronic sources of information in a way that augments rather than interferes with good communication. We move from:

Accessing electronic information both on the Internet and within the practice, whilst with the patient.

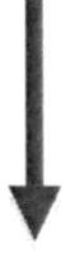

Using the computer, but not allowing the flow of the consultation to be disturbed as a result of becoming computer-focused rather than patient-focused

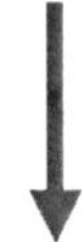

Using the data and information available from computer to increase patient understanding and enhance rapport.

Looking at each of the competencies in turn:

Uses the computer record and online information during the consultation.

The information revolution has meant that for large sections of society, i.e. those who have access to a computer and are happy to use it, obtaining electronic information is routine and expected. Not many years ago, patients were asked to come back when we had had the chance to 'look up' their condition. Nowadays, broadband, search engines and trustworthy sources of information make many such re-attendances unnecessary, except of course when we are trying to buy time!

We should know which websites are authoritative/useful and be able to access these easily.

Which types of website are useful to us?

These might include:

- Search engines e.g. Google
- Medical organisations: RCGP,BMA etc,
- Evidence-based medicine: NICE, Cochrane, Bandolier etc.
- Clinical guidelines: British hypertension Society, Society of gastroenterology etc
- Doctors sites: Doctor's net etc
- GP training sites: local vocational training schemes etc
- Journals and magazines: BMJ, BJGP etc
- Local organisations: primary care trust, LMC etc
- Patient sites

At this basic level of ability, we make use of the computer, but perhaps in a way that is not integrated with the consultation. As a result, communication may be adversely affected and the focus on the patient may not be maintained.

Uses the computer during the consultation whilst maintaining rapport with the patient.

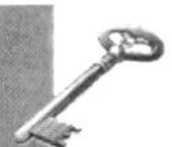

Because the patient-centred consultation is so central to the work of the GP, **this competency is felt by most educators to be particularly important in this performance area.**

To be 'competent', we have to integrate the use of the computer with the flow of the consultation, maintaining the focus on the patient and the problem rather than allowing a consultation to be focused on the use of the computer or on attending to the demands it generates e.g. to complete a template.

Several things can be done to help achieve this. Firstly, *fluency* with the use of the computer allows us to access data quickly, thereby reducing time spent away from communicating directly with the patient. *Positioning* the computer is important. If the screen is in the same direction as the patient, we do not need to turn the body away from the patient and eye contact can be maintained for longer. The downside is that it may be more difficult to use the screen as part of the consultation, looking at records or presenting data, graphs and photographs for the patient to look at and discuss.

It can often help to *be explicit* with patients about the use of the computer rather than hope that patients will find it acceptable. Mechanisms include acknowledging/ apologising that the computer may interrupt the flow of communication, *signposting* that the computer is about to be used, *explaining* what is being looked for or involving patients, perhaps by checking an entry or by inviting them to enter their own data such as smoking or alcohol consumption.

Patients are quick to notice if we are distracted. Therefore, when talking to the patient it may be better to give them full attention and show them that you are listening and not doing something else (like typing) at the same time. This encourages them to be more forgiving when the computer is used.

Patients regard the computer as being less intrusive if we can show how it helps us to improve their care. For example, we may show a hypertensive patient the recent trend in blood pressure readings in graphical form on the screen.

Computers make demands through their prompts and these can (and often should) be difficult to ignore. However, the prompts are unlikely to be on the patient's agenda and unless they are explained (e.g. 'for our records, I need to check whether you smoke') they will interfere with the consultation and may annoy the patient.

In terms of timing, some doctors reduce intrusion by entering their notes after the consultation rather than as they go along. However, even if our memory is good, this can sometimes be difficult to do because of technical factors. For example, if prescriptions are issued during the consultation but the notes are written later, the link between the problem and the medication may not be automatically created.

If notes are made during the consultation and patients can see the screen, rapport may be compromised if what is being typed does not accord with what the patient thinks was said. Some doctors also ask the patient to check the accuracy of the record that is being made. Doctors may therefore have to explain what is being written if the text could be misunderstood or might cause anxiety. This can happen for example when using abbreviations, when using alarming terms like 'heart failure' or when recording confidential or sensitive information.

Incorporates the computer records and online information in the consultation to improve communication with the patient.

This competency is high level because it demands fluency with communication and a sophisticated understanding of patient partnership. Let us consider this further with a brief detour.

This is a good place to consider why we collect information and what we use it for. TS Eliot famously asked 'Where is the wisdom we have lost in knowledge? Where is the knowledge we have lost in information? He was alluding to the fact that data has a purpose, which broadly speaking is to help us extract meaning that we can then use to make sound judgements. He was also illuminating a hierarchy from a low level of meaning (information) at the bottom to a high level of meaning (wisdom) at the top.

In communicating with the patient, we are continually interpreting data in order to extract meaning. Because we work in partnership with the patient to jointly derive suitable management options, it is important that both parties help each other to interpret the data and extract the meaning that it contains.

At the top of the hierarchy, Eliot mentions 'wisdom' which can be an off-putting term to some because of its connotations of philosophy and spirituality. However, in our medical context it is worth considering further because wisdom helps us to apply knowledge to practice and because of this, it has practical as well as philosophical relevance to our work as problem-solvers. The literature on wisdom suggests that an individual who exhibits wisdom:

- Knows a lot.
- Prefers to view problems from a broader long-term perspective.
- Sees things in context.
- Is flexible in adopting the multiple perspectives of multiple stakeholders.
- Recognises the uncertainty of life and the limits of their knowledge.
- Is prepared to be tentative or flexible in the kinds of solutions that they offer

Wisdom is therefore about being able to see information in a wider context, which in practical terms means trying to understand who or what might be affected by a problem and in what ways. In shorthand, we refer to this process as understanding the *implications* of a problem. Wisdom also requires us to think about which course of action might do the most good. To do this we must think about *ethical and social* considerations as well as medical ones. We can therefore see that wisdom is part of our holistic approach to patient care. Becoming wiser takes a long time because it requires us to have a lot of experiences of real-life problems, to sustain our motivation to learn the implications of problems (in particular, complex ones) and apply this growing insight to our professional judgement.

Let's now return to this competency, which is to do with making use of information to improve communication. We can now see that the reason for improving communication is in order to improve the *understanding* that doctor and patient have of the problem. This helps us to decide what information to look for and how to share it. For example, we may use information sources that *explain* rather than just inform patients. If our intention is to help patients to understand, it is helpful to use our *teaching skills* and think about the tools that we might use to get a message across. These might include information leaflets, diagrams and photographs. We may recommend books or programmes, give patients homework and encourage them to question us. To improve communication, we need to understand the patient's thoughts and preferences and again, the computer records can help. These may contain information about the past medical history, pre-morbid personality, the patient's preferences regarding medication, how they have responded to previous interventions and so on.

To help develop our communication skills, we could get feedback from colleagues watching the consultation or sitting in and (although this is rarely done) we could ask patients themselves what they thought of our attempts to inform/educate them and which techniques they found helpful or unhelpful. Try it sometime!

Needs Further Development	Competent for licensing	Excellent
Routinely records and codes each clinical contact in a timely manner and follows the record-keeping conventions of the practice.	Produces records that are coherent and comprehensible, appropriately and securely sharing these with others who have legitimate access to them.	Seeks to improve the quality and usefulness of the medical record e.g. through audit.

3

The third progression is specifically about good medical recordkeeping, which is the foundation of good medical care as well as the main evidence of it. We move from:

Making a clinical record, which may not be sophisticated but is produced routinely rather than sporadically.

↓

Making records that are cover the major areas, are understandable (e.g. with regard to the use of abbreviations) and are shared with those who need to know.

↓

Analysing the usefulness of records and trying to improve their quality.

Looking at each of the competencies in turn:

Routinely records and codes each clinical contact in a timely manner and follows the record-keeping conventions of the practice.

At this basic level, we need to demonstrate that we are reliable and can be trusted to make a record either at the time of the clinical contact or shortly thereafter. The record may be made after the patient has left the room, to avoid disrupting the patient-centred focus of the consultation. The clinical contact could occur in surgery, but may be a home visit, telephone consultation or internet contact.

Being reliable is critically important for two reasons. Firstly if the patient is given advice but no record is kept, a subsequent consultation will be disadvantaged. For example, the next clinician will not know if there were any significant findings or particular thoughts about differential diagnosis or follow-up. Also, an important pattern may take longer to be recognised, with implications for patient safety.

Secondly, if no record exists and something goes wrong, it can prove very difficult to defend medicolegally. Those looking at our performance may well regard poor record-keeping as being suggestive of poor professional standards in *other* aspects of our care. This may seem unfair, but experience shows that there often is a correlation.

You may wish to audit your notes, looking for: a record of the presenting problem, working diagnosis, some attempt to exclude important differential diagnoses, management plan, follow-up arrangements and use of appropriate computer codes.

Record-keeping conventions

Find out how the practice likes information to be recorded. For example, which codes are used and how do you find out which these are?

What are the templates that need to be completed? How are conditions recorded as being active or inactive?

How are drugs authorised for repeat prescription and how are these checked to minimise errors?

How are problems linked to medication?

What about letters that you need to write. How are these recorded/coded?

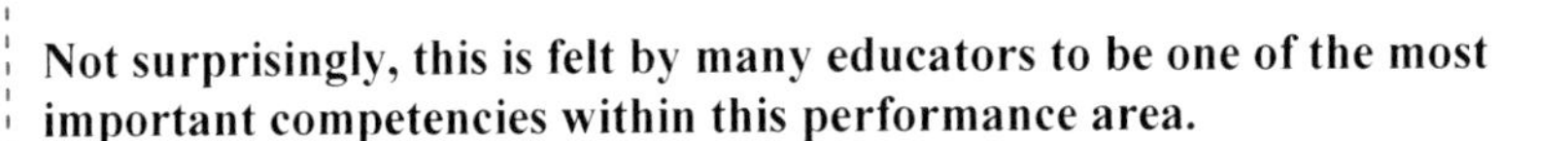

Produces records that are coherent and comprehensible, appropriately and securely sharing these with others who have legitimate access to them.

Not surprisingly, this is felt by many educators to be one of the most important competencies within this performance area.

It is said that a good medical record should *recreate the consultation*. In reality, this would probably produce essays! Although lengthy entries may seem to be better because they are fuller, they may deter other people from reading them. In addition, it may be difficult to pick out the important points from the background 'noise'. For example, although it may be important to write down certain significant negative findings (e.g. a lack of photophobia in patients with severe headache) lengthy lists of negative findings are unhelpful and obscure the salient points.

To be competent, the record should also be 'coherent and comprehensible' (see box on the next page)

For notes to be easily understood they should be written clearly, avoiding unnecessarily complicated technical language and only using abbreviations or shorthand phrases that are commonly understood. An additional factor is that patients often read their records, for example as they are being written in consultation or on request. This is an added incentive to avoid mystifying the record.

Doctors have a responsibility to keep records secure. Practically, this may mean that we take care to avoid putting records on screen where they can be seen by those who do not have legitimate access. For example, if we were to investigate the patient's background by looking at her husband's notes whilst she was in the room, we would have to ensure that she could not see the screen.

Records should also be shared with other clinicians involved in the patient's management where this is needed. For example, if a significant event has occurred such as a child protection issue, or if a referral has been made, the need to inform others will be obvious. Sometimes, sharing a record is needed in order to maintain good clinical care, for example when we go on holiday and another doctor is temporarily taking over the patient's care.

Seeks to improve the quality and usefulness of the medical record e.g. through audit.

At the excellent level, we may improve the medical record in a number of ways. For example, a formal audit of record keeping might be conducted to look at variation between clinicians in the records that they keep. This can act as a prompt for discussion.

Individual feedback may be (tactfully) given to colleagues when records are inadequate or incomplete such as when a computer prompt to 'check the patient's blood pressure when next seen' is left unattended.

Abbreviations can be a problem when they are not commonly understood, so an agreed list may be drawn up with a key to the abbreviations. These abbreviations may also cover aspects of examination and management.

The technology of the computerised record can also enhance its usefulness. For example, computer macros might be used to enter standardised text such as the advice given for a viral URTI, or to produce a standardised prescription, for example for Helicobacter eradication.

More complex macros can be used e.g. to generate a summary of the patient's diagnoses, repeat medication, allergies and most recent consultations that can be used when referring a patient or admitting a patient to hospital.

Coherent notes

This means that notes should be **orderly, logical and consistent**. The computer lays down an orderly structure by virtue of the subheadings used, through which the clinician is guided when making a record.

Being logical means that relevant information in relation to the problem is sought and recorded. Therefore, an ESR would seem to be a relevant investigation for a patient with headache, but an MSU would not.

Being consistent means that our thinking, as seen from the notes, is justifiable on the basis of the available information both within this consultation and from previous consultations that relate to the same problem.

13 Management: Community orientation

This competency area is about the management of the health and social care of the practice population and local community.

This section of the competence framework demonstrates better than almost any other, how the mindset and concerns of GPs are different to those of other specialists. For the trainee, this section presents a particular challenge because, other than in the section on resource management, it does not build on much of our previous training. Having said that, the context is not unfamiliar as undergraduate and pre-specialist training increasingly provide exposure to aspects of community medicine.

This area takes us beyond the focus on the patient and gets us to think about the wider community. There are three separate but related themes which build progressively on each other as this chapter shows:

- Understanding the features of the local community
- Understanding the nature and availability of local healthcare resources
- Managing resources, in particular the tension between the needs of individual patients and the wider patient community

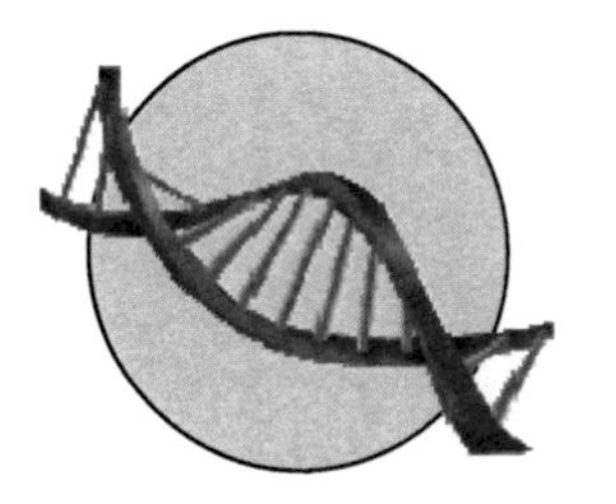

Which aspects of our DNA, our deeper features, are prominent in community orientation? If we look back at the competencies for the 'Management' section (see page 117), we see that **problem-solving skills** are particularly important.

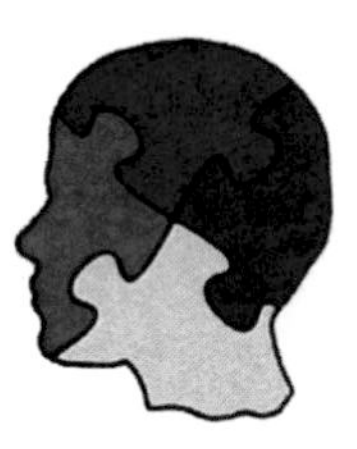

Joined up?
See p14

Needs Further Development	Competent for licensing	Excellent
Identifies important characteristics of the local community that might impact upon patient care, particularly the epidemiological, social, economic and ethnic features.	Applies an understanding of these features to improve the management of the practice's patient population.	Uses an understanding of these features to contribute to the development of local healthcare delivery e.g. service design.

1

Discussion point: the inverse care law

The inverse care law was first described by Dr Julian Tudor Hart in 1971. It states that 'the availability of good medical care tends to vary inversely with the need for it in the population served.' This law is often quoted because availability, access to and use of services are thought to vary in accordance with this law.

Those who need healthcare least are said to use services such as the treatment of disease and health promotion more frequently and more effectively than those with the greatest objective need.

Sometimes people in need are 'excluded' by the system. Try looking at those who are 'exception reported' from QOF and check the reasons for this.

The first progression is about the importance of understanding the local community and how doctors tailor their services to meet the community's needs. We move from:

Having an understanding of those features of the local community that make it different from other populations.

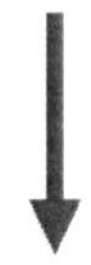

On the basis of this understanding, being able to improve the way current services are provided.

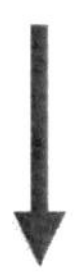

Developing existing services and designing new ones to improve local healthcare

Looking at each of the competencies in turn:

Identifies important characteristics of the local community that might impact upon patient care, particularly the epidemiological, social, economic and ethnic features.

GPs don't just treat *patients*, but provide healthcare to a local *population*. Getting to know the features of the local community is therefore more than just getting to know the patients and we can improve our insight by considering the community from different, but interrelated, perspectives.

Our aim as GPs is to maximise the health of our local population and to do this, we need to understand the factors that influence health, the degree of influence that we have over these factors and how we can best improve community health within the available resources. Of course, this is not just *our* responsibility. Social services and education have a large part to play and in future, particularly through greater involvement in the commissioning of health services, GPs will be more actively involved in community health.

The word picture identifies some key features of the population, which we will now discuss.

1. Socioeconomic

Let's start by considering the relationship between socioeconomic factors and health. Of the 'characteristics of the local community' mentioned above, this relationship is particularly important and addressing it is part of what many practitioners most value about working in the NHS. Let's consider this in more detail.

The NHS was established in 1948 to address the inequality in health care services. It was set up as a service that was free at the point of use, was responsive to local needs and had a fairly even geographical spread across the country. The idea was that all citizens should receive the same high standard of care. As a result of the state-funded system, doctors no longer clustered in the most prosperous areas, because their livelihood was no longer dependent upon the patient's ability to pay. Also, patients of all socioeconomic classes were able to get the care of a practitioner when they (the patients) felt it was required. The power of these principles cannot be underestimated. Ask yourself: how would you feel and what would you do if you had to turn away patients could not pay your bills? This happened frequently before the NHS.

Why is access to healthcare important? There are some significant factors that we should be aware of. The first is that there is a clear correlation between position on the socioeconomic scale and the health that might be expected. This can be difficult for people who are more privileged in life (including doctors) to appreciate.

The evidence shows us that:

Together with inequalities in mortality, inequalities in *morbidity* contribute to large differences in the number of years of healthy living that might be expected.

Typically, persons with high socioeconomic positions live more than 10 years longer in good health than those in the lowest positions.

The *relative* as well as the absolute gap is important. Life expectancy data in England indicated in the early 21st century that since 1997 the relative gap in life expectancy had increased between England as whole and the 20% of local authorities with the lowest life expectancy. There were also differences between genders; in men the relative gap increased by nearly 2%, in women by 5%.

Health inequalities are mainly caused by greater exposure in lower socioeconomic groups to material, psychosocial and behavioural (smoking, alcohol consumption, nutrition) risk factors.

Studies looking at deprivation and the quality of primary care services show that the quality of care (e.g. glycaemic control in diabetes and influenza immunisation uptake) falls with increasing deprivation.

There is a social gradient in health according to income, occupation, education and parents' social class.

Tip: thinking about health and socioeconomic factors

You may be asked about this relationship in knowledge tests, but you should also think about the practical application of this knowledge.

Of the social factors listed, which do you feel you have an influence over? How would you apply this influence in dealing with a patient's problem? We have a clear role in managing addiction and stress…but what else?

Now think about your own practice. Which factors are particularly important in your own community? How would you find out?

What if anything have you done in your practice to address these issues? What do you think is a good use of your time and what is not?

Whose responsibility is it to join up health and social services? Can you think of any practical small scale project that is a good example of this in your community?

So what are the main social factors that impact upon health?

- Stress (modifying factors being control ,predictability, degree of support, threat to status, presence of outlets)
- Inadequate housing
- Early life (the effects of early development last a lifetime: a good start in life means supporting mothers and young children)
- Social exclusion
- Work control
- Organisational justice
- Job insecurity
- Social support
- Unemployment
- Addiction (Individuals turn to alcohol, drugs and tobacco and suffer from their use)
- Food
- Transport

The single assessment process (SAP): an example of integrating health with social factors

This is an example of how policy developments have recognized and reflected the importance of taking both medical and social factors into account when thinking about health. The SAP in this example relates to the health of older people. The table overleaf shows questions developed by the East Birmingham Primary Care Trust.

It's worth looking through the questions. Do any surprise you? Some look at social factors that are not frequently asked about (e.g. do you feel safe?) and others challenge our assumptions about the elderly (do you have any sexual concerns?).

Housing is a major social factor, but interestingly this questionnaire takes a more sophisticated look by asking not about housing itself, but about the effects of inadequate or inappropriate housing. Which do you think these questions might be?

SAP Questionnaire	
MAINTAINING A SAFE ENVIRONMENT	**COMMUNICATION**
o Have you any history of falls? o Are there any hazards in the home? o Are you able to summon help? o Are you able to self medicate? o Do you have any memory problems?	o Have you have any problems with your eyesight, hearing or speech?
BREATHING	**EATING AND DRINKING**
o Do you have a persistent cough? o Do you have any difficulties or discomfort breathing?	o Do you have any difficulties with eating, chewing or swallowing? o Have you had any weight loss? o Do you have any problems preparing meals or shopping or feeding yourself? o Do you have adequate cooking facilities?
ELIMINATION	**PERSONAL CLEANSING AND DRESSING**
o Do you have any problems passing urine? o Do you have any problems with your bowels? o Do you have adequate toilet facilities? o Do you have a catheter or stoma? o Do you use any laxatives? o Are you able to get to the toilet/ commode?	o Do you have any skin problems including eczema, pressure sores and leg ulcers? o Can you wash dress and undress without assistance? o Do you have any carers/ statutory or voluntary?
MOBILISING	**CONTROLLING BODY TEMPERATURE**
o Do you have any problems mobilising e.g. walking unaided, climbing the stairs, walking outside? o Do you have any pain or joint stiffness?	o Is there heating in the house – upstairs / downstairs? o Do you have adequate bedclothes?
SOCIAL/LEISURE	**PSYCHOLOGICAL**
o Do you have any financial problems? o Do you have regular social contact? o Do you have difficulty getting to public services? o Do you have any support services?	o Are you in any pain? o Do you feel down / low? o Have you any concerns over your condition? o Do you feel safe inside / outside your home? o Do you have any sexual concerns?
SLEEPING	**HEALTH PROMOTION**
o Do you have trouble sleeping or take night sedation? o Do you go to bed at night?	o Do you smoke? o Do you exercise regularly? o Do you drink alcohol? o Have you had a flu jab? o Have you had any screening? e.g. breast, cervix, prostate, cholesterol, BM, BP. o Are you concerned about your weight?
CARERS NEEDS	
o Do you have any problems getting out? o Do you have any support? o Do you feel able to carry out the care?	

Tip: ethnic and cultural factors

Look at the patient profile for the practice. Ethnicity data may be held by the practice or by the primary care organisation. Find out which are the significant ethnic minorities. Do they have any special needs by virtue of ethnicity or culture?

Talk to the clinicians in the practice and find out if they experience any particular difficulties in dealing with this population. How do they modify their approach? This might include their consulting style. Does it also include any clinical tailoring?

Do some research to find out whether the ethnic minority population is at risk of any particular conditions. Are the GPs aware of these? Are any steps taken to screen for these? If you feel such steps are appropriate, try suggesting how the practice could go about this. This will provide excellent evidence of competence in this first progression.

Remember, it's *applying* your understanding that matters. It may not be possible to demonstrate that an actual improvement has occurred as a result of your actions, but showing some initiative and taking action that might later lead to improvement is what is needed.

2. Epidemiological and ethnic/cultural factors

Having considered the socioeconomic factors, let's think about the epidemiological ones that might have an influence on community health. The curriculum suggests a number of examples and it is worth remembering that some of the community are affected by more than one of these factors.

- Environmental and genetic factors affect the prevalence of metabolic problems e.g. Diabetes is more prevalent in the UK in patients of Asian and Afro-Caribbean origin.

- Hypertension is more common in patients of Afro-Caribbean origin and their responsiveness to standard hypertensive treatment is different than in Caucasian patients.

- Hyperuricaemia is more common in prosperous areas and is associated with obesity, diabetes, hypertension and dyslipidaemia

- Environmental and geographical factors influence the prevalence and treatment of cancers. For example, mining communities are at particular risk of respiratory pathology.

- Cultural and ethnic factors will influence treatment, for example Jehovah's Witnesses will not take certain forms of medication. These factors may challenge our approach to ethical issues, for example ritual circumcision in certain communities.

In clinical management, we need to exercise caution because the majority of evidence-based guidelines do not include ethnicity or socio-economic status as risk factors. For example, we know that algorithms to assess the risk factors for cardiovascular disease underestimate the risk in south Asian populations. Additionally, many studies are conducted in secondary care and are not always generalisable to primary care populations.

Applies an understanding of these features to improve the management of the practice's patient population.

Why is it important to go one step further and make use of this understanding? The reason is powerfully summed up in the following statement:

What good does it do to treat people's illnesses and then send them back to the conditions that made them sick?

Changing the conditions is therefore vital. If this is not done, we achieve little more than fire-fighting rather than preventing future combustions from occurring.

Changes may be instigated *externally*. GPs are often involved in implementing health policy and in the coming years, there will be increasing emphasis on addressing obesity, smoking cessation and alcohol at population level. Efforts with smoking cessation therapy have proved successful initially, although there are concerns that without continued vigilance, population improvements may relapse.

GP practices have already been highly effective at reducing health inequalities, in particular through improving access to specific services. For example, differences in cervical cytology uptake rates narrowed markedly in the 1990s and GP practices are now routinely achieving the target of > 80% uptake. Here are a number of other examples of situations in which practices have been instrumental in improving health by applying their understanding of the features of the local population:

With stroke, enough is known about the risks of the disease to be confident that a systematic assessment of risk of all people aged 40–74 would be clinically and cost effective.

Male life expectancy in Birmingham has been improved through primary care by:

- targeted check-up offers to high-risk patients in 12 priority wards
- offering screening in community venues and
- offering heart checks in community pharmacies in target areas.

Better access to health promotion services has been developed for people with a learning disability, who are often unaware of the service and have difficulty with making the arrangements to come.

Alternatively, the initiative for changes may arise *internally*. For example, advances in medical science may lead to GPs looking at their current practice with new eyes. Because resources are limited, we usually target treatment to achieve maximum efficacy and our knowledge of population factors can be vital. If we don't have this knowledge, auditing the patient population can allow a profile of an 'at risk' group to be identified. To illustrate this, there are new drugs to manage chronic gout and this may prompt us to look at the epidemiology of the condition.

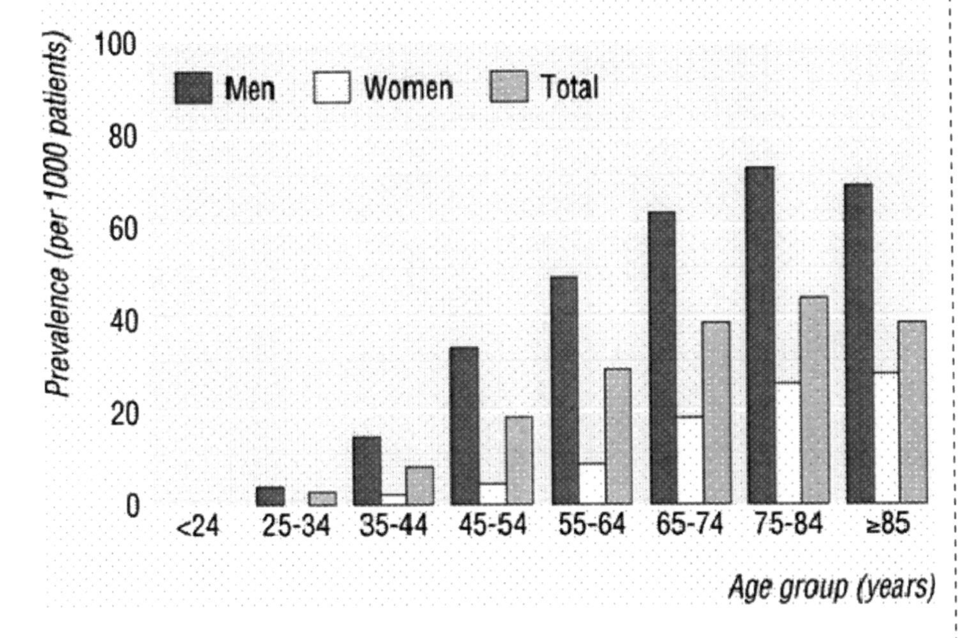

The histogram shows how the prevalence is very much higher in men, particularly from middle age onwards. On the basis of this, the practice may decide to review the treatment of middle aged men either opportunistically as they come into surgery or by inviting them.

Uses an understanding of these features to contribute to the development of local healthcare delivery e.g. service design.

Just to remind you that this competency is *above* the level required for licensing. It's importance is likely to increase as GPs take more active role in modifying and developing services and we can see how this competency builds upon the previous two.

A great deal is already going on with the development of integrated care pathways and the provision of near-patient services that were previously only available in secondary care. Here are some more examples of how GPs are delivering primary care in new ways:

In some communities, new premises are being built that provide primary care GP services alongside specialist clinics, for example for people with long-term medical conditions.

An alternative is to build centres that have well-being and social care services bolted on to clinical services such as diagnostics. Centres may have community beds and in this IT age, even a hub for 'tele- monitoring' of patients who are cared for at home.

Building community hospitals is an old idea that is coming around again, using them as hubs that link with home-care monitoring and support.

Needs Further Development	Competent for licensing	Excellent	
Identifies important elements of local health care provision in hospital and in the community and how these can be appropriately accessed by doctors and patients.	Uses this understanding to inform referral practices and to encourage patients to access available resources.	Uses an understanding of the resources and the financial and regulatory frameworks within which primary care operates, to improve local healthcare.	**2**

Whereas the first progression is about understanding the people that make up the local community, the second is to do with the resources that are available to them. We move from:

Knowing what resources are available both in the community and in hospital and how these can be accessed

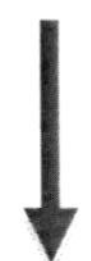

Using this understanding to make targeted referrals to the appropriate agency and where relevant, educating patients as to what is available and how to access healthcare resources.

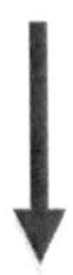

Beyond accessing what is currently available, using our influence to improve the local provision of resources in line with what the population needs.

Tip: knowing what is available

In order to do your job effectively, you will probably need to keep a diary or address book in which the important contact details are logged.

You may also wish to add information on whether or not the patient can self-refer to these resources.

This list of contacts is good evidence of having achieved the first level.

Looking at each of the competencies in turn:

Identifies important elements of local health care provision in hospital and in the community and how these can be appropriately accessed by doctors and patients.

This basic level is mainly about information gathering and there are two stages involved. **Firstly** we need to find out what hospital and community services are available. There may be specialist hospitals such as oncology and children's hospitals as well as district general or teaching hospitals. In the community, there will be a number of healthcare services provided by other members of the primary health care team such as health visitors, district nurses, midwives and community mental health workers.

Less commonly, there may be chiropodists and community physiotherapists. It is worth being aware of the roles and availability of paid carers, respite care and the services offered by local voluntary and statutory agencies.

In between community care and hospital care, there may be specialist outreach nurses such as diabetic and epilepsy liaison nurses, who can give specialist advice and support and can usually be contacted directly by sufferers.

You should already know the opening hours of your practice, including any extended hours that it offers. You will also need to find out how out-of-hours care is provided and how patients can access GPs and other providers of emergency care such as A&E, NHS direct and walk-in centres.

Secondly, you need to find out for whom these services are available and how they can be accessed by doctors and possibly directly by the patient.

As we saw in the first section in this chapter, social services are intertwined with health. It is therefore important to know how social services can be contacted by doctor and by patient.

Uses this understanding to inform referral practices and to encourage patients to access available resources.

As with many of the progressions, the basic level deals with understanding the issues whereas ‘competence’ is reached when we are able to apply what we have learned.

Assessors will look particularly closely at referral practises. Good referral practise partly means that the problem has been appropriately defined and that we have appropriately decided that it is beyond our sole management. However, it also means that the inquiry has been appropriately directed.

Because patients' problems can often be managed in a number of ways, 'encouraging patients to access available resources' may mean advising them about a range of people and resources that are available. For example, the curriculum teaches us that for visually impaired adults, we might recommend:

- RNIB talking books for the blind
- low vision aids
- financial support

Also, because GP care is holistic, we think of the patient in their own context which means that when we offer help, we think about the needs of the patient's family and carers as well as the patient. When it comes to resources, carers are frequently overlooked.

Many self-help groups for patients with significant/chronic conditions are good sources of support for carers and can often signpost other useful resources that you may not be aware of.

When you have offered such help, which might include advising about websites or giving a patient information leaflet, it is worth recording this in the medical record. This will help others involved in the patient's care to see that wider forms of help have been offered and will also provide evidence of your competence in this area.

Tip: evidence of competence from referral audit

To be competent, you should be able to show that your referral practises are 'informed'. Therefore, a quick audit of referrals, preferably including referrals to community resources as well as hospital clinics, should provide good evidence for your portfolio.

In the audit, look for the reason for referral and evidence of appropriateness (for example, that the referral was accepted and dealt with rather than redirected or sent back).

If you look further, you can use the same audit to provide evidence of other competencies such as clinical management and team working. It is entirely appropriate for one source of evidence to be used for multiple purposes in this way.

Uses an understanding of the resources and the financial and regulatory frameworks within which primary care operates, to improve local healthcare.

This descriptor of excellence shows how we apply knowledge of the healthcare system rather than just our biomedical knowledge, to improve the health of a whole community of people rather than individual patients. To do this, we need to understand the system well enough to know *where* it needs to be changed and *how* change can be brought about.

This depends upon a number of things including knowing where the faults lie in the current service, the characteristics of the local population and what they need, what they expect (which may not be what they clinically need), what is feasible, allowable and what is cost-effective. As you can see, this is a complex calculation!

Making such improvements can occur at practice level, where it is mostly within the control of a few people and can happen quickly. Improving the services for the disabled through better access to the premises, or for deaf patients through better messaging systems such as a visual display, are two examples. The need for this might be prompted by knowledge of the legal frameworks within which primary care operates, which for the examples just given is the Disability Discrimination Act.

At locality level, making improvements is a much larger team-based exercise and to demonstrate this 'excellent' competency, we need to show that we are contributing to such exercises. For instance, there may be a need to allow GP access to imaging such as MRI scanning for orthopaedic problems, for example instability of the knee. This could be developed collaboratively between GPs, orthopaedic surgeons and radiology departments and an appropriate protocol produced. Recommendations could also be made by the group as to how the new service could be audited to check that it is meeting the needs that have been identified and is being used appropriately and cost-effectively.

Needs Further Development	Competent for licensing	Excellent
Identifies how the limitations of local healthcare resources might impact upon patient care.	Optimises the use of limited resources, e.g. through cost-effective prescribing.	Balances the needs of individual patients with the health needs of the local community, within the available resources.

3

The third progression builds upon the previous two. Having understood the nature of the local population and the current availability of resources, we move from:

Understanding what the resource limitations are and how doctors have to work around these locally

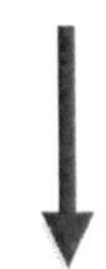

Managing resources, being cost-aware, and where possible, cost-efficient.

More widely, being aware of the tension between serving the individual and serving the local community and trying to achieve a justifiable balance between the two.

Looking at each of the competencies in turn:

Identifies how the limitations of local healthcare resources might impact upon patient care.

This theme, although separate, is related to the previous two. Once we have found out about the local resources, we have to understand the local population to know how the limitations in resources might impact upon their care. At one level, the impact will apply nationally as for example with the limitations imposed by guidelines such as NICE. At another level, the local community might be affected by factors that are related to their specific needs. For instance, a lack of local translators might severely affect the healthcare of a non-English-speaking community.

Sometimes, national restrictions can have a differential affect on communities because of local factors. Restricted access to anti-obesity drugs may therefore

Tip: service redesign

Even if you are not yet able to demonstrate the 'excellent' competency, you can learn a great deal by joining in any service initiatives that your practice is part of.

Ask the GPs and practice manager about the practice development plan/business plan. Identify an area of service improvement and speak to the lead clinician or manager in the practice.

If you can, try to observe how the process is carried out, perhaps by sitting in at one of the relevant meetings.

Questions: If you were asked to make a suggestion, which area of service would like to improve? Why would this be your priority?

affect socio-economically deprived communities (where the incidence of obesity is higher) more than affluent communities.

The implications of rationing: developing your insight

Try taking a topic that interests you and talking it through in a group, **addressing each of the following factors**:

- Why and how rationing occurs
- The intended and unintended consequences
- The way in which quality of healthcare is gauged (which is not just quantitative but also includes measures of quality of life)
- The political dimension and the ethical principles (particularly autonomy and justice) that are challenged by the rationing issue.

Discussion: identifying local limitations in resources

Start close to home and find out from doctors and nurses in your practice where they think the limitations lie. A good place to start is to think about cutbacks in service and the impact that this had. For example, has the practice lost services that it used to provide, such as chiropody, physiotherapy, extended district nursing services? Have these been missed and if so by whom and why?

Beyond this, what services do local practitioners feel should be provided, but are not yet available? Again, what impact does this lack of service have on the local community? Do practitioners feel that this adverse impact is any worse locally than it would be nationally? If so, why? This question will help to gauge the relative importance of local factors.

Moving to locality level, try to find out what the priorities of the local commissioning body are. What limitations are they trying to rectify and why?

You can make a reflective note of your findings, which will be of interest to the practice and will be excellent evidence for your portfolio.

There are ongoing national debates about rationing. The curriculum suggests that you should be able to, for example:

- Describe the rationale for restricting certain investigations and treatments in the management of cardiovascular problems e.g. open access echocardiography, statin prescribing.
- Describe the rationale for restricting certain investigations and treatments in the management of skin problems e.g. prescribing of retenoids, access to phototherapy.
- Evaluate the effectiveness of the primary care service you provide from the male patient's point of view.
- Evaluate the arguments for and against a national screening programme for colorectal cancer.
- Discuss the rationale for restricting referrals for upper gastrointestinal endoscopy in the management of dyspepsia.

Optimises the use of limited resources, e.g. through cost-effective prescribing.

This competency is thought by assessors to be particularly important. You will notice that the word 'optimises' is used. This is because we are not simply talking about rationing, which often has negative connotations of cost-cutting, but about making the best use of resources and thereby ensuring that the greatest good is done for the greatest number of people (a utilitarian principle). Very often, making the best financial use of resources is not in conflict with producing the optimum management plan. For example, the curriculum teaches us to:

1. Recognise the place of simple therapy and expectant measures in cost-effective management, whilst ensuring that the patient's condition is adequately monitored.
2. Prioritise referrals accurately so that people with minor conditions don't delay/compromise the care of those with more serious conditions.

3. Avoid investigations or treatments that are unlikely to alter outcomes, so that the availability of these resources (e.g. imaging methods) is optimised.
4. Deal with situational crises and manipulative patients appropriately, without resorting to inappropriate investigation or referral.

Balances the needs of individual patients with the health needs of the local community, within the available resources.

The nub of this complex competency is understanding that we have responsibilities to individual patients *and* to wider communities. In a sense, one patient's gain is potentially another one's loss given that resources are finite and always will be.

To demonstrate this competency, we must be able to explain and justify the decisions that we make by showing that we recognise the tensions and have a rational way of approaching them. Probably the most important abilities that we need are to show sensitivity and awareness for the problems that rationing creates, particularly in the human dimension and to avoid prejudice and undue bias in trying to reach a compromise.

The word 'resources' should be widely interpreted. We are not just talking about finances, but about services, including our own time. Therefore, making optimal use of resources means thinking about *time* spent with patients as well as investigations, referrals and prescribing costs. The curriculum illustrates these points by teaching us that we need to:

- Give morally relevant reasons for decisions that balance individual patient needs with the needs of the wider community.
- Provide more time in the consultation in order to deal more effectively with some people, for example those with sensory impairment or learning disabilities.
- Consider the workload issues raised by patient problems, especially the demand for urgent consultation, and the mechanisms for dealing with this.

Note that the curriculum points out that 'balancing resources' means that we must also plan to give some people more resources than others. Such people are often, by virtue of their condition, less able to speak up for their needs and in these situations, part of our role as doctors is to act as their advocate.

Tip: demonstrating the optimum use of resources

You could readily demonstrate cost-effective prescribing by showing that you prescribe generically and by recording situations in which you chose a more cost-effective drug or avoided a more costly formulation, such as a modified release drug where this wasn't necessary.

Now look at the four numbered principles in the text. Try to produce evidence of these, particularly of the first three as the opportunity for these occurs frequently.

Examples from the range of areas discussed in this box will be ample evidence for the portfolio.

Demonstrating the ability to balance resources

Important evidence of this ability will come from situations where you are aware of a conflict between opposing demands. It is helpful to think of these situations as being **' significant ethical events'** and in line with this, write a significant event analysis arising from personal reflection and discussion with peers. The essence of demonstrating this competency is being able to show that ethical principles have been used to inform the resource decision and that you have tried to recognise personal bias and where relevant, compensate for this.
Evidence might also arise from multisource feedback provided you have involved your colleagues in discussing your ethical dilemmas.

Let's consider another aspect of 'resources'. Quite often, when doctors talk about 'demanding patients', what they mean is *'inappropriately* demanding' patients! Managing such patients is difficult and emotionally draining. Part of the balance that we have to consider is the one between giving the patient what they want and confronting the patient, with the risk of a time-consuming complaint and damage to our emotional health. Time lost with complaints is an important loss of medical time that could be spent on patient care. On the other hand, not dealing with such an issue may simply store up problems for ourselves or colleagues in the future and is not fair to the majority of patients who don't shout for attention. In managing this we have to remember that *our* health is also an important resource that is finite and should be used with care.

In the next and final chapter on 'Management', we will consider how we manage ourselves well enough to maintain our performance.

14 Management: Maintaining performance, learning and teaching

This competency area is about maintaining the performance and effective continuing professional development of oneself and others

This is the longest chapter in the book, which gives you some idea of its importance. Although the profession worries a great deal about performance, it is telling that it is not uppermost in patients' minds. This may be partly because patients don't know quite what to look for, but it is also because they assume that keeping up to date and maintaining our performance will be so important to us that they can take it for granted. Do we as a profession and you as a doctor live up to this assumption?

Maintaining our medical performance is no different to maintaining our physical or mental performance. Think of it as 'health promotion' but with the added dimension that we are doing it partly for ourselves but mostly because others may come to harm if we don't.

What does this mean in practice? Performance, like health promotion, is not just about having good intentions; anyone can give up smoking once they've been told they have lung cancer. Maintaining performance is about respecting its importance to those dependent upon us, having the commitment to do something regularly and having a mechanism for doing so.

The *mechanism* is vital, because it underpins performance. This section is part of the 'Management' section of this book because it concerns our ability to *manage ourselves by monitoring* our performance, learning and development in all relevant areas, and therefore maintain the capacity to keep working throughout our careers at a sufficiently effective and safe level.

Why do we need a mechanism? This is because no matter how good our self-awareness might be, we can't rely upon it as the only trigger that prompts us to learn. 'Patient harm' is like an iceberg. By the time we become aware of the tip, most of the harm has been done. By having a mechanism to monitor ourselves and keep up to date even when we are not prompted to do so, we keep the 'Sea of performance' warmer and don't allow so many icebergs to form.

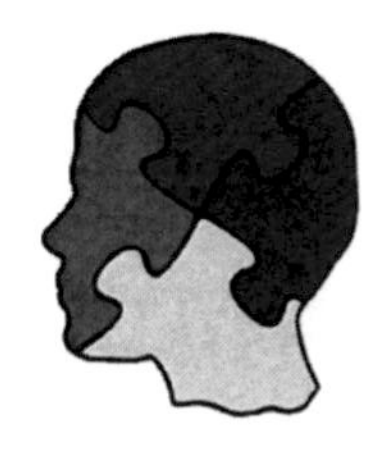

Joined up?
See p14

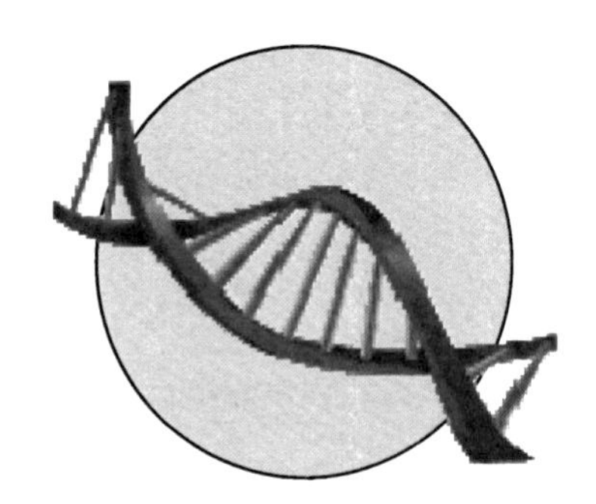

Which aspects of our DNA, our deeper features, are particularly important in maintaining performance, learning and teaching? If we look back at the competencies for the 'Management section (page 118-120), we see that learning and personal development skills are particularly important, followed by team working skills.

Let us look at the competencies that are being tested in this section:

Needs Further Development	Competent for licensing	Excellent	
Accesses the available evidence, including the medical literature, clinical performance standards and guidelines for patient care.	Judges the weight of evidence, using critical appraisal skills and an understanding of basic statistical terms, to inform decision-making.	Uses professional judgement to decide when to initiate and develop protocols and when to challenge their use. Moves beyond the use of existing evidence toward initiating and collaborating in research that addresses unanswered questions.	1

This first competency progression is about how we engage with evidence-based practice and illustrates how we move from:

Understanding the importance of accessing the available evidence, and doing so routinely. In addition, knowing what question to ask, where to look and doing so effectively and in a timely manner.

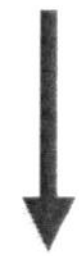

No longer simply *accepting* what is written , but using critical appraisal skills to decide whether what is suggested is valid and important enough to act upon.

Using critical appraisal and evidence-based skills to challenge recommendations that do not appear valid. Additionally, spotting the gaps and suggesting where protocols need to be developed or research needs to be initiated and being prepared to play a part in this process.

Looking at each of the word pictures in turn:

Accesses the available evidence, including the medical literature, clinical performance standards and guidelines for patient care

Evidence-based medicine is the cornerstone of modern medical practice and an important part of maintaining performance is to make routine use of it. Firstly, a word of warning. As we have seen elsewhere in this book (page 105), the evidence upon which recommendations (particularly therapeutic) are made, often come from secondary care settings where patients used in studies may not be representative of those seen in primary care. For example, many of the early recommendations on antidepressant therapy came from studies on inpatients with severe depression who were selected because they not have significant additional problems such as anxiety or alcoholism. However, in primary care, most patients who are treated for depression have mild/moderate forms of the condition and usually have significant co-morbidity. Mixed anxiety/depression is very common as is alcohol abuse, which can both be a cause and a result of the condition.

This does not mean that evidence should be disregarded, but the example shows that we need a sophisticated understanding of evidence-based medicine in order to apply the recommendations appropriately and challenge them when inappropriate, rather than following them unthinkingly.

The curriculum identifies the importance of being aware of relevant national guidelines. If you can't recall whether a guideline exists, a quick Internet search is often worth doing as a check. To make any sense of the outcome of a search, we need to know which guidelines are more authoritative or trustworthy than others. We will consider this in more detail later. Here are a few examples of what the curriculum recommends regarding searching EBM, the areas where evidence is important and key guidelines we should be aware of and use:

Searching

Be able to use decision support to make their interventions evidence-based e.g. Cochrane, PRODIGY, etc.
Search the internet for medical and scientific information including MEDLINE

Demonstrate understanding that evidence needs to be gathered from the most appropriate, rather than the most readily available source. You should be able to determine whether the evidence is sufficient and rigorous enough to be analysed in the context of a patient.

Guidelines

ENT: diagnosis and treatment, particularly with respect to ENT interventions of dubious efficacy. Having an evidence- based approach to antibiotic prescribing, to prevent the development of resistance e.g. otitis media.
Respiratory: BTS / SIGN guidelines on asthma management, the NICE guidelines on COPD management
Neurology: NICE guidelines on epilepsy diagnosis and management
Oncology: Knowledge of cancer treatment trials and how to inform patients about their participation
Musculoskeletal e.g. the NICE guidelines, RCGP low back pain guidelines, SIGN guidelines
Cardiovascular: NICE guidelines, British Hypertension Society Joint Committee recommendations, National frameworks and quality markers
Metabolic: Describe the role of particular groups of medication in the management of diabetes (e.g. antiplatelet drugs, angiotension converting enzyme inhibitors, angiotensin-II receptor antagonists, and lipid lowering therapies). Describe the key research findings that influence management of metabolic problems (e.g. UKPDS, DCCT
Mental health: adopting a critical and research-based approach to practice is particularly important in mental health, where evidence on effective treatment may be of poor quality.

Discussion point: obtaining evidence of 'accessing the available evidence'

You should be familiar with the relevant search engines/ websites that are commonly used. If the practice has not done this for you, you may wish to add some to your Internet 'favourites'.

Try to involve patients when you do searches during the consultation by showing them what you are looking for and discussing your interpretation of what you read. This is good practice in helping to develop your critical appraisal skills, and (if appropriately explained) enhances patient understanding and trust.

Patients are generally more confident of doctors who check by looking things up than those who appear to know it all. In addition, accessed material is sometimes useful to print off for the patient.

Assessors may see evidence of 'access' by observing your consultations.

Other issues

Being aware that recommendations may change across the four countries of the UK.

In the modern world and particularly medicine, we are bombarded with information so a key skill in 'accessing the available evidence' is knowing which articles are worth taking the time to read and which should be ignored. This process is sometimes called 'literature triage' and it can save a great deal of time to have a rational way of approaching it. Although the original article is not shown here, we can illustrate some of the principles of critical appraisal through an analysis of a paper in the following section.

Suppose we were interested in developments in the contraceptive pill and we saw an article on the combined pill, Yasmin, published in the drug and therapeutics bulletin. The manufacturer suggests that this pill has positive lifestyle effects, particularly on weight, acne and quality of life. How could we decide whether the article was worth reading in depth?

Is this article worth taking the time to review in depth? ***A 'stop' or 'pause' answer to any of the following should prompt you to question seriously whether you should spend the time to review the article critically***		
Is the article from a peer-reviewed journal? *Articles published in a peer-reviewed journal have already gone through an extensive review and editing process.* Yes: the drug & therapeutics bulletin is an independent review from the consumers association. Peer review indicates that the article has been assessed before publication. I am more likely to trust the results. Because the drug & therapeutics bulletin is independent, their opinion is impartial, unlike publications sponsored by drug companies and special-interest groups who will wish to put their own spin on the results	Yes (go on)	No (stop)
Is the location of the study similar to mine so the results, if valid, would apply to my practice? The review does not talk about the populations in this detail. The difference between populations would be important to know in certain situations (for example, lifestyle advice in Kensington would not be the same as in Barnsley!). However, Pill advice is likely to be the same in any community-it is not particularly different for different ethnic groups, for example. For this reason, the fact that populations are not defined more explicitly doesn't really matter.	Yes (go on)	No (pause)
Is the study sponsored by an organization that might influence the study design or results? *Read the conclusion of the abstract to determine relevance.* See notes above. The important thing is that the organisation is impartial.	Yes (pause)	No (go on)

Could this information, if true, be important to the way I practice?		
I have to decide whether the information is important to me, i.e. whether it might have an effect on the way I practice. Equally, the condition should be considered important by my *patients*. However, they may not always be aware of what might be important to their health. In this situation, I might be influenced to read this article as my patients are already asking about this pill, so it is obviously important to them. If papers relate to areas of practice that I don't have responsibility for, it is probably not worth my while reading further although it may be worth making a colleague aware.	Yes (go on)	No (stop)
Is the intervention feasible and available to me? Sometimes, changes are recommended but the treatment that is being suggested is not available. For example, if Yasmin was not prescribable then this article would only be of academic interest. In this instance, I have responsibility in the family planning clinic and am able to make recommendations about treatment to my colleagues. Therefore, it is worth my while reading further.	Yes (go on)	No (stop)
Will this information, if true, require me to change my current practice? Yes. However, I have to remember that research must first be *statistically* significant. If it is significant (meaning that the beneficial effects are not just down to chance alone), I have to then decide whether it is also *clinically* significant. For example, any claims for lack of weight gain have to be put into perspective. Small amounts may not justify a change in treatment. If the results ***are*** clinically significant, I also need to think about whether they are *cost-effective* and whether the new treatment would be *acceptable* to patients. For example, Yasmin may have problematic side-effects of its own.	Yes (go on)	No (stop)

Judges the weight of evidence, using critical appraisal skills and an understanding of basic statistical terms, to inform decision-making.

Most doctors recognise the importance of critical appraisal, but many feel insecure about using these skills. With many of the best available guidelines, a critical appraisal process has already been carried out and so the need for practitioners to do so independently, becomes less necessary. However, as we have discussed above, doctors routinely access a wide range of material some of which is dubious value and most of wish has not been triaged. In addition, patients increasingly come with 'evidence' which without some knowledge of critical appraisal, we are in a poor position to evaluate, use or recommend.

In the previous section, we looked at how to decide whether an article is worth studying in depth. Let's continue this thought process by now considering whether the Yasmin article that we read is worth acting upon.

The table overleaf shows that although involved, the process of critical appraisal is not double-Dutch and it does have a useful outcome. Being able to reason in this way will become increasingly important as we become more involved in how finite resources are used at local level.

Tip: developing critical appraisal skills and obtaining evidence

Critical appraisal can seem abstract and therefore of low priority. The secret to developing the appropriate skills is to learn them in the appropriate practical context rather than simply from the books. That way, you will see their value and develop the *motivation* to want to be competent in this area.

Most practices have access to a prescribing adviser and these colleagues often have practical critical appraisal skills that they can share with you. Make time to discuss the issues they are working on in the practice and find out how critical appraisal helps them to give the appropriate advice.

Additionally, you could use the table shown in the text as a pro forma to work through, for example, with information on a new therapy. The *prescribing adviser could also provide evidence of your ability* that you could use for your portfolio.

Some practitioners get together to do a journal club, perhaps as part of a wider clinical meeting. Try taking an interesting article along and presenting a brief critique using the relevant parts of the table as a guide.

If the article passes the initial screening discussed previously, proceed with the following critical assessment by reading the methods section. ***A 'stop' answer to any of the following should prompt you to question seriously whether the results of the study are valid and whether you should use this new drug***		
Is the study a randomized controlled trial? a. How were patients selected for the trial? b. Were they properly randomized into groups using concealed assignment? At the top of the hierarchy of evidence in EBM is the randomised controlled trial. This is placed highest because the greatest efforts are taken to reduce bias. From the general population, patients are divided into those who receive the intervention and those who do not, by a process called randomisation. This reduces the bias that might occur if researchers decided who got the new treatment and who didn't (perhaps based on who they thought might benefit and who would not). Articles at the bottom of the hierarchy (case reports) take no steps to reduce bias and therefore are less likely to be acted upon, because they are anecdotal. There are exceptions to this when, for example, case reports suggest an important outcome such as mortality or severe morbidity following the use of a drug. The Yasmin report selects randomised controlled trials only, so I am more likely to take notice of the recommendations. The numbers involved were large (a good thing as this makes the results more likely to be definitive). The studies were *not* designed to test 'well-being' defined by the manufacturers as 'no associated weight gain, a positive effect on pre-menstrual symptoms and skin condition'. In fact, the studies were designed to look at inter-menstrual bleeding. This makes me suspicious that the manufacturer's claims that Yasmin produces greater well-being, may not be well-founded.	Yes (go on)	No (stop)
Are the patients in the study similar to mine? European study. This probably reflects my own population, as the number of ethnic minority groups in my locality is not high. This may not have been the case if I was working in an inner-city practice	Yes (go on)	No (stop)
Was everyone involved in the study (participants and investigators) 'blind' to treatment? Two published non-blinded trials were used. Blinding (where researchers and patients were not aware of who was receiving which treatment) would have been better in reducing bias.	Yes	No
Were the groups treated in the same way (aside from the experimental intervention)? We don't know. For example, some patients may have been given dietary advice to reduce weight. The weight loss noted in the study may have been due to this rather than Yasmin. The reviewers also comment that weight was measured by patients themselves (not by the researchers). The women were aware of which pill they were taking. This might have had an effect. For example, if they were expecting the new pill to help with weight reduction they may have mis-reported their weight	Yes	No

Are the results clinically as well as statistically significant? Were the outcomes measured, clinically important? Although not as medically important as, say, cardiovascular effects, the other outcomes are very important to patients and are therefore clinically important to me. There were problems with the outcomes, as follows: Weight was self-reported. The amount of weight loss was not clinically significant although it was statistically significant. Acne was not defined, so it is hard to say how much clinical improvement occurred. Again, how pre-menstrual symptoms were reported is not defined. The report doesn't state how severe the symptoms were, therefore we cannot say how clinically significant they were. Quality of life was measured by questionnaire. How this group was selected is not made clear. Only 10% of the potential study population actually completed a questionnaire. This is too small to be a representative sample. Cardiovascular effects were reported by levels of cholesterol and triglyceride rather than clinical outcomes, which would have been more meaningful.	Yes	No
Were there other factors that might have affected the outcome? The studies were not designed to look at lifestyle effects. The researchers would probably not have thought carefully about how weight, skin condition and quality of life should be assessed. This is reflected in the fact that there are many problems (listed above) with how these factors were actually analysed. The manufacturers are seeking to use information from trials retrospectively to make a claim that is probably unjustified from the results.	Yes	No
Are the treatment benefits worth the potential harms and costs? No, as the drug and therapeutics reviewers make clear in their conclusion	Yes	No

The curriculum guides us that we need to understand the fundamentals of statistics such as the p value, incidence, prevalence, NNT (Number needed to treat), sensitivity and specificity of a test.

This terminology relates to *quantitative* studies. Of course, many questions don't have numerical answers and particularly in general practice where patient outcomes are complicated and not easily measurable, research often needs to be qualitative. *Qualitative* research in general practice may appear 'woolly' and even frustrating, because it produces grey rather than black and white outcomes. However, taken cumulatively, this type of research can guide us best because it can address the questions that most concern us in the community. For example, in the treatment of otitis media, we are more interested in whether fever, days off school and long-term complications such as deafness are reduced, than in whether a particular bacterium has been eradicated.

We've now considered how doctors can access the evidence and judge its weight. The point of this information, as this competency states, is to inform decision-making. In doing so, it's important not to use EBM in isolation. We must take into account other factors that influence the decision, which include the patient's health beliefs and values.

The curriculum speaks of recognising the use of value-judgements to complement the evidence-based approach. This dual approach is explained in the curriculum statement 'clinical ethics and values-based practice' in more detail. Here are some practical examples of how the two concepts work together in helping doctors to arrive at the best decisions:

- Having an awareness of the range of values that may influence a patient's behaviour or decision-making in relation to his or her illness
- Knowing how to integrate knowledge of patients' values with the relevant scientific evidence and clinical experience to achieve the best outcome for the patient
- Having the ability to recognise the ethical issues raised by public health programmes and develop appropriate approaches to their implementation
- Being aware of tensions between science and politics of screening, which may colour the recommendations being made.

Uses professional judgement to decide when to initiate and develop protocols and when to challenge their use.

As we discovered, the critical appraisal process allows us to see when research guidance is or is not appropriate or applicable to practice. Once we have adequate skills to critique documents well enough, we are in a position to achieve this level of excellence.

Increasingly, the documents that most powerfully influence (some would say, constrain) medical management are in the form of guidelines or protocols. Although these documents look authoritative, it's important that we do not simply accept them at face value, but question their validity in primary care.

Guidelines have been defined as

'Systematically developed statements to assist practitioner decisions about appropriate health care for specific clinical circumstances'.

The ***benefits of guidelines*** are to make the process of decision-making more objective and transparent, to systematically introduce evidence-based decision-making, and to act as an assessment yardstick for use by patients, doctors and supervisors.

The ***problems with guidelines*** are that they may not be objective but reflect expert opinion, they may inhibit innovation and cause practices to 'regress to the mean', and that they may not be applicable at local level or within our own practices. Once again, there is a systematic way of critiquing the guidelines, and when we do so the following areas should be carefully thought about:

Choice of topic
Are the guidelines dealing with an important-enough topic? The topic should concern a high-volume, high-risk or high-cost issue. There may be large or unexplained variations in practice. There should be potential for improvement with the likelihood that there will be interest from professionals and benefits for patient care.

Objective
The nature of the health problem, the subjects and setting as well as the providers of care should be stated.

Options
The various approaches to dealing with the problem that were considered in the development of the guidelines should be discussed.

Outcomes
The health and economic outcomes used to compare the clinical practice options should be stated.

Evidence
How the evidence was gathered, selected and collated and by whom, should be known.

Benefits, Harms, Costs
These should be considered from the perspective of both the provider and the patient.

Validity and Applicability
- How strong is the evidence on which the guidelines are formulated?
- Are the guidelines applicable to general practice (or were they developed for use in secondary care?)
- Are the guidelines comprehensive? They should deal with most clinical eventualities. To be useful, guidelines should help us manage patients who fall outside the clinical mainstream.
- Are the guidelines feasible? Can I implement them in my practice, do I have the resources and would they be acceptable to my patients?
- Have the guidelines been validated by external review or clinical testing?

Sponsors
Is there a conflict of interest (such as pharmaceutical sponsorship) that may influence the applicability of these guidelines?

Authors
Look for objectivity. Paradoxically, experts are less objective at appraising evidence in their own specialty than in someone else's.

The closer to home the development of the guidelines has been, the more likely you are to implement them, both because you may have greater ownership of the development process and because the recommendations may be more applicable to your own population.

Moves beyond the use of existing evidence toward initiating and collaborating in research that addresses unanswered questions.

In general practice, unlike secondary care, research is not yet embedded as a routine part of our activity. This seems paradoxical considering the concerns we have about transferring hospital based evidence to primary care settings. However, the hope is that the situation will change in the coming years in line with changes to GP training. Certainly, there is no shortage of important research questions that we could ask!

This competency, at present in the 'excellent' category, describes how we show and apply our intellectual curiosity. To get into this mindset, try to move beyond asking yourself 'What?' and instead ask 'Why?' and 'What if.....?'

Although the vast majority of us will not become researchers, we can fulfil a vital function by facilitating research in primary care so that the evidence-base of the future is tailored to our needs rather than being imported from less suitable contexts. For example, we might allow bone fide researchers access to our patients to seek consent for studies or else we might participate in multi-centre trials on, for example, the treatment of asthma.

Establishing links with the research community also means that we can generate questions that the researchers may choose to investigate.

Needs Further Development	Competent for licensing	Excellent
Routinely engages in study to keep abreast of evolving clinical practice and contemporary medical issues.	Shows a commitment to professional development through reflection on performance and the identification of and attention to learning needs. Evaluates the process of learning so as to make future learning cycles more effective.	Systematically evaluates performance against external standards, using this information to inform peer discussion. Demonstrates how elements of personal development are related to the needs of the organisation. Uses the mechanism of professional development to aid career planning.

2

The second competency progression is thought by many educators to be the most important in this area of performance. It relates to the mechanism and effectiveness of learning and continuing professional development. The word pictures describe how we move from:

Putting time aside to keep up-to-date and doing so routinely

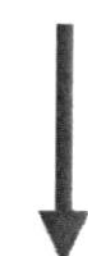

Beyond keeping up-to-date, being able to identify learning needs, act upon these and progressively become a more effective independent learner

Using learning in a wider context as part of the mechanism for maintaining standards, contributing to the performance of the organisation and helping career progression

Looking at each of the word pictures in turn:

Routinely engages in study to keep abreast of evolving clinical practice and contemporary medical issues.

At this basic level of performance, we have to have a systematic way of keeping up-to-date. Note that the competency is not about demonstrating clinical competence, but about showing that we have a *mechanism* of doing so.

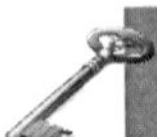

Shows a commitment to professional development through reflection on performance and the identification of and attention to learning needs.

These attitudes and skills are so important that without them, safe practice is not possible, which is why they are highly rated by trainers and assessors. Changes to contemporary practice are always occurring and without a CPD mechanism, even doctors who at the time of licensing are well above average, will quickly become significantly underperforming. CPD may therefore be analogous to walking up an escalator that is going down. Stop moving and you go down, walk faster and you go up. A minimum is perhaps to walk fast enough to stay at the 'good enough' level.

It's a fact that competence decays over time without some mechanism of rectification. It also a fact that ***competence decays much more quickly than confidence***, which means that you may *feel* that you are up-to-date even when colleagues recognise, or the data suggests, that you are not.

This competency refers to two elements. Firstly, the need to reflect upon performance, which means that there must be some way in which we collect information on our performance (particularly the feedback of assessors) and try to evaluate what this means. How does this accord with our own self-assessment? The difference between what others think of us what we think of ourselves, is a measure of our **insight**. Provided that we are being honest when we make our self-assessment, the *gap* tells us something important about ourselves. Once again, doctors who underperform in the eyes of others, tend to rate themselves more highly than others do or in other words, their insight into their own performance is relatively poor.

The reason that this is important is that in independent practice, doctors depend upon good insight in order to pick up on *minor* aberrations and deal with these before they become major ones. Minor aberrations (i.e. small differences between what they do and what is generally held to be acceptable) are unlikely to be picked up by colleagues, which is why insight, having an effective CPD mechanism and the motivation to improve are critically important. If these are not in place, problems will not be recognised until they are large, by which time patient safety may already have been compromised and the corrective action that is needed may be significant. We might summarise this point by saying that insight is better than hindsight!

Additionally and importantly, the problems that we have to grapple with in primary care are complex and don't have their answers in textbooks. Insight is therefore vital in order for the right questions to be asked after which an effective learning mechanism is needed for them to be translated to answers that can help patient management.

Developing insight is important, but how do we attend to our learning needs? This is the second part of the competency. The schemata shown overleaf was produced for use by independent practitioners when writing their personal development plans (PDP) for NHS appraisal. The principles apply just as well to trainees, who, being NHS employees, are also required to undertake appraisal. With trainees, learning plans are reviewed more frequently and the amount of objective evidence of performance is rather greater than is usually available for independent practitioners,

Tip: evidence on keeping up-to-date

The evidence is not so much that you have put time aside for studying, but that through case discussion etc, you are seen to be in touch with recent developments and suggested changes to current practice.

Remember that 'keeping up-to-date' relates to all aspects of medical practice, including changes to service delivery, changing political and societal expectations and so on.

Health care and GP services are frequently in the news and it's a good idea to become familiar with one source of news such as a GP magazine, the health section on news websites etc. so that you know the hot topics of the day.

Events occur so frequently in general practice that even a week away from base can make you feel out of date!

which makes CPD easier to demonstrate during training than afterwards. In the schemata, the acronym **SMART** stands for Specific, Measurable, Achievable, Relevant and Time-Bound.

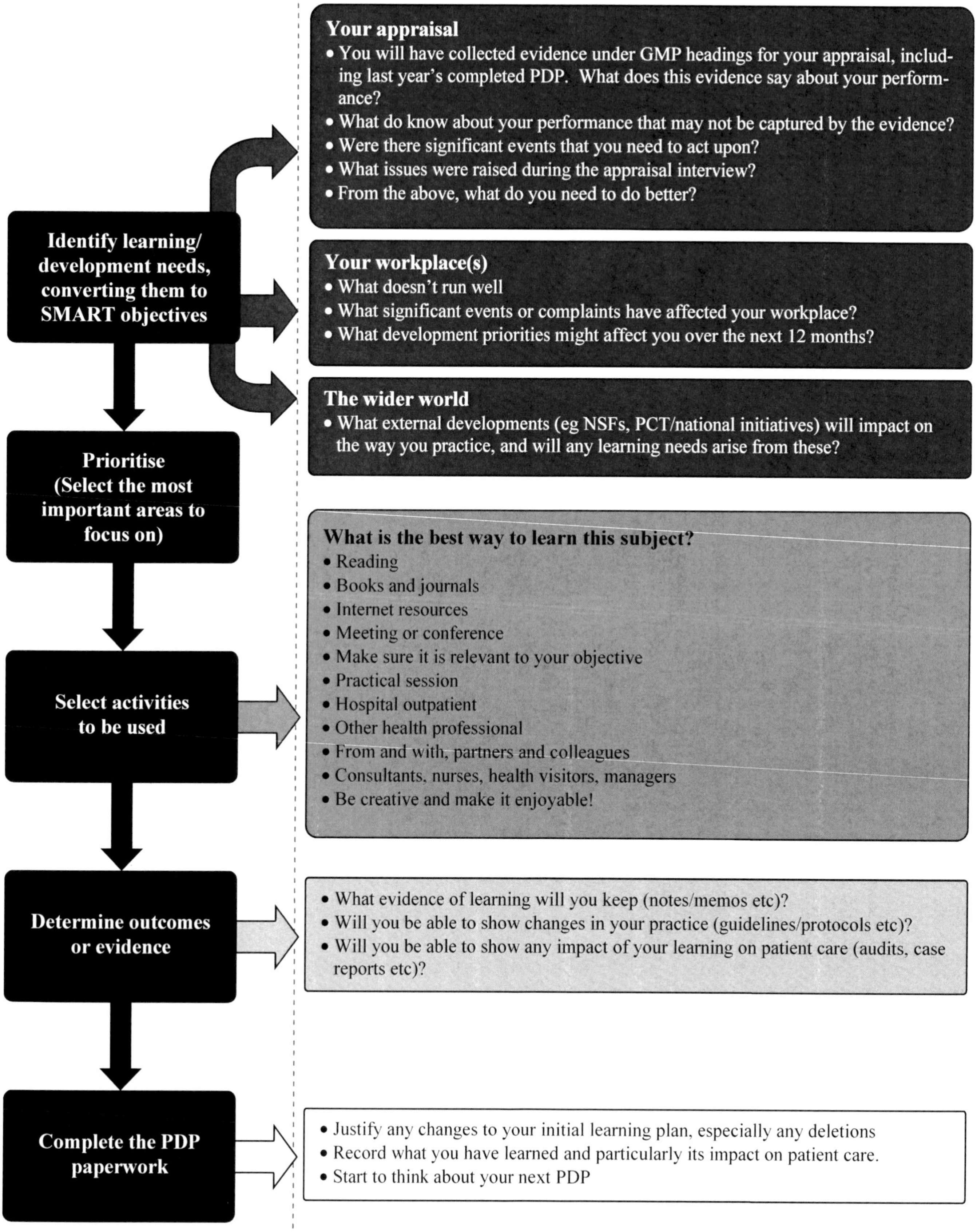

Identify learning/ development needs, converting them to SMART objectives

Your appraisal
- You will have collected evidence under GMP headings for your appraisal, including last year's completed PDP. What does this evidence say about your performance?
- What do know about your performance that may not be captured by the evidence?
- Were there significant events that you need to act upon?
- What issues were raised during the appraisal interview?
- From the above, what do you need to do better?

Your workplace(s)
- What doesn't run well
- What significant events or complaints have affected your workplace?
- What development priorities might affect you over the next 12 months?

The wider world
- What external developments (eg NSFs, PCT/national initiatives) will impact on the way you practice, and will any learning needs arise from these?

Prioritise (Select the most important areas to focus on)

Select activities to be used

What is the best way to learn this subject?
- Reading
- Books and journals
- Internet resources
- Meeting or conference
- Make sure it is relevant to your objective
- Practical session
- Hospital outpatient
- Other health professional
- From and with, partners and colleagues
- Consultants, nurses, health visitors, managers
- Be creative and make it enjoyable!

Determine outcomes or evidence

- What evidence of learning will you keep (notes/memos etc)?
- Will you be able to show changes in your practice (guidelines/protocols etc)?
- Will you be able to show any impact of your learning on patient care (audits, case reports etc)?

Complete the PDP paperwork

- Justify any changes to your initial learning plan, especially any deletions
- Record what you have learned and particularly its impact on patient care.
- Start to think about your next PDP

The competency requires evidence of **reflection**. This can be produced in free text form, either unstructured or using a structured reflective template such as the one shown in this chapter on page 167.

Evaluates the process of learning so as to make future learning cycles more effective.

The concept here is that doctors not only learn, but they learn how to 'learn more effectively'. They do this in a number of ways as suggested by the evaluation questions in the form shown below.

DEVELOPMENT PLAN -- EVALUATION
How did you identify your learning needs for this PDP, and what other methods might you include in your next PDP?
Which objectives were easiest to achieve and why?
Which objectives were most difficult to achieve and why?
Which were the most valuable learning activities and why?
Which were the least valuable learning activities and why?
In what ways have you been able to apply your learning to patient care?
What benefits to your patients do you feel have occurred as a result of your learning?
Are there any learning needs that you wish to carry forward to your next PDP?

Tip: evidence on learning

Reflection on performance is vital as this is the main evidence of insight. Assessors will gauge this through your learning plans, including the PDP that is produced for NHS appraisal.

The schemata shown on p160 should be used so that a rational approach to learning can be demonstrated. The PDP *evaluation questions* should also be answered as these show evidence of targeted reflection and also help you to become a more effective learner.

Systematically evaluates performance against external standards, using this information to inform peer discussion.

This competency is categorised as 'excellent' because it requires us to look for external standards against which to compare our performance and to have both the motivation and mechanism for doing so systematically. Additionally, the outcomes of this process are used for discussion with colleagues in order to inform personal development. To do all this requires us to have a high degree of professionalism, self-awareness, initiative and the ability to constructively accept criticism. These attributes are not acquired quickly or without discomfort.

The training system requires young doctors to be judged and to act upon feedback, which on occasion they may perceive as criticism. Doctors in independent practice are in a different relationship with their peers and work in an environment where autonomy is greater, formal supervision is absent and mutual respect is just as important and just as fragile. In these circumstances, being open about performance and being able to accept and act upon criticism is hard because relationships and reputations are at stake. Nevertheless, it is important that all doctors do so and the cultural change to bring this about will be catalysed by doctors who are currently in training.

To achieve this competency requires us to look for relevant external standards. This means comparing performance against what the profession regards as adequate rather than what *we* feel is good enough. These standards may be available through quality frameworks such as QOF or through the medical literature.

Where no such objective standards exist, comparison against peer performance is an appropriate and accessible alternative. Except in very small practices, this can be easily done by comparing performance of individuals with the performance of colleagues. Revalidation requires doctors to demonstrate evidence of *personal* performance. Practice audit where the data is presented so as to allow individual and group performance to be displayed is an ideal way of achieving this.

Tip: evidence of tie-in with the needs of the organisation

This can be achieved by showing that some of your personal objectives lie within the practice professional development plan.

Alternatively, you could comment on how your personal need was related to the development of the practice.

The competency speaks of using this information to inform peer discussion. This could occur on a one-to-one basis or alternatively, practices may use attributable audit data to prompt group discussion. As long as this is not done on a 'name and shame' basis, such discussions can be productive and can motivate practitioners to change behaviour.

Demonstrates how elements of personal development are related to the needs of the organisation.

Although 'learning for learning's sake' is valuable, as our job is to deliver a service, it is appropriate for some of our learning to be directed to the needs of the practice/organisation. This does not mean that every element of learning is targeted to a pre-defined practice need, but it does mean that it would be inappropriate if *none* of it did so.

Practices vary in how they define their needs. Many needs arise spontaneously and are acted upon opportunistically. In other more predictable situations, there may be a formal process of producing a practice development plan/business plan that formulates mutually agreed needs and sets objectives over a specified timescale. Some practices formally align the learning activity of the practice members with the needs of the organisation through a practice professional development plan (PPDP) which has the advantages of concentrating the group's efforts on the practice's needs and of allowing resources to be obtained to meet the learning needs, some of which may be common to several members of the practice.

Uses the mechanism of professional development to aid career planning.

Career planning is often neglected by practitioners. When we move into different areas of responsibility or make significant changes to our working lives, this often happens without planning, simply because the opportunity arises. This is not *wrong*, but the notion that we can plan head for significant changes, and thereby make it easier for ourselves, is often overlooked. Reflective practitioners can learn as much about themselves as about their learning needs through the process of professional development. This information is precious because it can help us to recognise what motivates us, where our strengths and weaknesses lie, what our capacity for change might be and how effective we are in achieving our goals.

Given the right circumstances, for example through discussion with an appropriate person such as a mentor, these insights can be used to plan for significant changes in our careers and our lives. Some of these changes are predictable, such as the years spent as a parent, as the head of a practice or the years in retirement. Even for such commonplace but important life changes, discussion about the implications and how best to prepare can be enormously valuable.

Needs Further Development	Competent for licensing	Excellent
Changes behaviour appropriately in response to the clinical governance activities of the practice, in particular to the agreed outcomes of audit and significant event analysis. Recognises situations, e.g. through risk assessment, where patient safety could be compromised.	Participates in audit where appropriate and uses audit activity to evaluate and suggest improvements in personal and practice performance. Engages in significant event reviews and learns from them as a team-based exercise.	By involving the team and the locality, encourages and facilitates wider participation and application of clinical governance activities

3

The third progression shifts the focus away from the individual and considers the practice-wide measures taken to improve quality and protect patient safety and how these can inform our learning. We move from:

Responding to the outcomes of audit, patient safety incidents and significant event reviews.

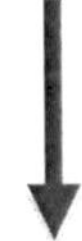

No longer acting in isolation but participating in and initiating audit and significant event reviews and making suggestions about personal and practice improvements based on these.

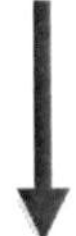

Using these performance review activities in a wider context to improve health services in the locality.

Looking at each of the word pictures in turn:

Changes behaviour appropriately in response to the clinical governance activities of the practice, in particular to the agreed outcomes of audit and significant event analysis.

The competencies in the NFD column are extremely important, because they underpin our ability to monitor and maintain performance when we are no longer being closely supervised through training.

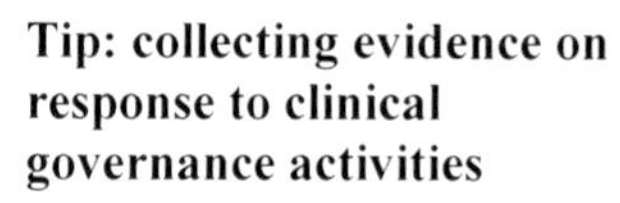

Tip: collecting evidence on response to clinical governance activities

Doctors who are temporary members of a team will have difficulty in obtaining information from many clinical governance activities, because data on their performance may not be routinely collected.

Look at the list and highlight the ones that you feel you could obtain information from.

Discuss your thoughts with doctors/managers early on as they may be able to help you collect information, for example by adjusting computer data gathering systems to collect information on your referrals.

If audits are taking place, find out how your activities could be included in the analysis. Make a note of your engagement with governance activities such as health and safety training.

Your response to this information can be shown by a subsequent data collection or through activities in your learning plan.

The first competency requires us to respond to the clinical governance activities of the practice. Clinical governance (CG) is a framework of accountability that governs and promotes the efforts an organisation makes to continually improve quality. The first requirement is to understand what the CG activities of the practice are. Any process that promotes quality of care and can be evaluated, is a CG activity. The most important are audit and significant event analysis, but there are a range of CG activities that can give feedback on the performance of individuals, such as:

- Incident reporting system
- Risk assessments
- Infection control
- Prescribing review
- Conformation to NICE guidelines
- Participation in clinical audit
- Fraud policy
- Equality and diversity training
- Management of records and patient information
- CPD in the practice such as clinical meetings/journal clubs
- Compliance with research governance processes
- Confidentiality and consent systems
- Complaints procedures
- Health and safety protocols in the practice

The competency requires us to 'change behaviour appropriately'. This means that if performance is adequate, changes may not be needed. However, as insight is always being developed and confirmed, it is good practice to discuss our performance with more senior colleagues and then decide whether changes are needed or not. The outcomes of significant discussions provide good evidence for the portfolio.

'Changing behaviour' also involves demonstrating a commitment to improvement. Audit and significant event analyses are specifically mentioned because these are important sources of information and are usually discussed in a team-based exercise from which action points arise. We would normally follow through these action points as part of our commitment to the team and the service.

Recognises situations, e.g. through risk assessment, where patient safety could be compromised.

Patient safety, as a concept, is becoming increasingly prominent and is now explicitly addressed as a major section of Good Medical Practice. Before discussing this competency, let's consider patient safety in more detail.

Patient safety is defined by the National Patient Safety Association (NPSA) as a process by which an organisation makes patient care safer. **This should involve**: risk assessment; the identification and management of patient-related risks; the reporting and analysis of incidents; and the capacity to learn from and follow-up on incidents and implement solutions to minimise the risk of them recurring.

How widespread is the problem? It has been estimated that around 10% of patients admitted to NHS hospitals have experienced a patient safety incident, and that up to half of these incidents could have been prevented.

For patient safety to be improved, there are two widespread myths that need to be scotched. These are:

The **perfection myth**: if people try hard enough, they will not make any errors;

The **punishment myth**: if we punish people when they make errors, they will make fewer of them.

Errors are inevitable because health care is complex, recommendations are constantly changing, people are human and make mistakes and no system is ever 100% reliable. This is not an argument for complacency, but the focus of patient safety needs to be clearly stated. The best way of reducing error rates is to target the underlying systems failures, rather than take action against individual members of the team.

The NPSA suggests seven steps to patient safety:

Step 1 Build a safety culture
Step 2 Lead and support your staff
Step 3 Integrate your risk management activity
Step 4 Promote reporting
Step 5 Involve and communicate with patients and the public
Step 6 Learn and share safety lessons
Step 7 Implement solutions to prevent harm

We can see from this that it is important to assess the practice's safety culture, perhaps by conducting a survey. For example, do team members feel able to talk about their concerns and report incidents without fear of recrimination?

The curriculum suggests that in addition to being aware of the concept, we need to acquire some specific skills, for example we should be able to:

- Describe the tools that can be applied in risk management and patient safety issues e.g. those accessible from sites such as www.saferhealthcare.org.uk and medical indemnity sites.
- Describe the basic principles of human error.
- Describe the basic principles of risk assessment.
- Demonstrate how to compile a simple risk matrix.

Risk assessment involves collating information on incidents that the practice becomes aware of. There are three types of incidents that should be reported:

- incidents that have occurred;
- incidents that have been prevented (also known as near-misses);
- incidents that might happen.

To learn the most we can from patient safety incidents, we should apply Root Cause Analysis (RCA) or Significant Event Audit (SEA) techniques.

These are techniques to review a patient safety incident to find out what, how and why the incident happened. They pinpoint areas for change, and they prompt recommendations for sustainable solutions that reduce the chances of the incident happening again. Further information on the RCA can be obtained from

http://www.msnpsa.nhs.uk/rcatoolkit/course/iindex.htm

Tip: looking for evidence on response to change

It may not be possible for change to occur quickly, but you should have plans and a reasonable timescale.

Evidence can arise from debriefing, MSF as well as from future data collection.

If trainees do not take action even when the need for this has been discussed, there may be other issues, for example difficulty in understanding the need for improvement, difficulties with time management, poor organisation skills or (more worryingly) poor attitude in not accepting the need for change.

Tip: collecting evidence on patient safety awareness

This competency requires us to show awareness of safety issues. Evidence can arise through case discussion, where we may be asked to identify areas in which things might go wrong and safety might be compromised.

The range of areas is extensive, for example risks inherent in inadequate diagnosis, management and follow-up, risks that arise through poor teamwork (especially communication) and risks attributable to patient behaviour.

Additionally, our behaviour such as incident reporting or participation in clinical governance activities, shows our awareness of safety.

Likewise, those who actively seek information on errors, perhaps by asking to be informed when things go wrong, are demonstrating a solid understanding of this competency.

At this basic level of performance, our focus should be on recognising the *range* of areas in which things might go wrong. In particular, we should understand that risk is multifactorial and things go wrong because a number of suboptimal circumstances come together to cause a near miss or actual patient harm. The *sources* of these problems are not just ourselves and the practice, but may include colleagues in the community or hospital, communication and data reporting systems and sometimes, the behaviour of patients themselves. Even if the factors that give rise to a particular patient safety incident are recognised, not all of them may be amenable to improvement.

Learning to recognise the range of factors allows us to make better safety netting arrangements. To take a simple example, we may tell a patient at the time of urgent outpatient referral to contact the practice if they have not had an appointment or a letter of acknowledgement within a defined time period. At a more sophisticated level, we may routinely look in the medical records to see if the presenting problem links with previous consultations, so that an important emerging pattern is not missed. For example, previous presentations with hoarse voice, discomfort on swallowing and occasional dry cough may not be recurrent URTIs but may be the early signs of malignancy.

Participates in audit where appropriate and uses audit activity to evaluate and suggest improvements in personal and practice performance.

This is the first of the 'competent' descriptors. We have now progressed to a stage where we do not respond in isolation to quality issues but see ourselves as part of a mutually-dependent team. Excellent performance in one team member cannot be made up for by suboptimal performance in another; i.e. we are only as good as our weakest link. For example, suppose an excellent practice nurse triaged a call from a patient with an acute blistering rash on the right shoulder and decided that a GP consultation was needed. On speaking to the nurse, we decided to prescribe a cream rather than see the patient, who later turned out to have shingles complicated by neuralgia. The latter could have been prevented with prompt antiviral medication had the patient been examined.

This competency refers specifically to audit activity. It still remains important for us to understand and implement the audit cycle. However, because of automated data collection, audit activity against certain national standards such as QOF occurs on a continual basis. Therefore, rather than waiting for an occasional audit to be performed, we have a wealth of information that can be used to continually profile our performance. Data can arise from a number of sources of which audit is one of the most important (see page 168).

To show competence, we should look at audit activity and suggest (where appropriate) improvements at a personal/practice level. QOF is not person-specific and therefore if there are areas of concern, these could be addressed by raising awareness in the practice and/or by looking in detail at the performance of individuals to see if the problem is specific or widespread. Sometimes, this is not necessary as, once the problem is identified, individuals may know from knowledge of their own behaviour whether there is need for change. Audit can be particularly useful where individuals are not aware of a problem because of lack of information, lack of insight or (rarely) denial.

Although many clinical markers exist in QOF, there are many other areas of personal and practice performance that will not be addressed through automated systems. In particular, we become aware when changes in clinical management are proposed or reminders about best practice are given. These can prompt an ad hoc audit, as can significant events in practice life.

When audits are prompted in this way, doctors can reflect upon the outcomes and consider whether changes are needed and following these, when to look for improvement. The following structured reflective template assists this process and provides good evidence for the portfolio both for training and for appraisal.

This competency mentions our ability to 'suggest improvements'. This means that we must not only correctly identify significant deficiencies in performance, but should be capable of making sensible suggestions about improvements. For example, the **suggestions should be:** relevant to the problem, feasible to undertake given the available resources, acceptable to those who are affected (including the patients to whom they apply) and preferably have measurable outcomes so that the degree of improvement can be gauged.

Data collection/audit structured reflective template
Name of doctor: GMC No:
Measurement/audit title: Date of data collection/audit:
Reason for choice of measurement/audit:
Audit findings:
Learning outcome and changes made:
New audit target:
Final outcome after discussion at appraisal: (Complete at appraisal considering how your outcome will improve patient care)

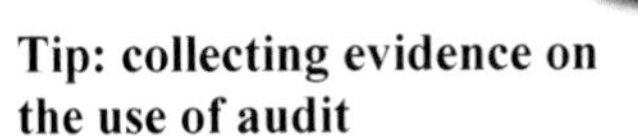

Tip: collecting evidence on the use of audit

You should be able to demonstrate that you are aware of the audit that goes on in practice and you should show that you learn from the audit outcomes.

You can show evidence of this by using tools such as the structured reflective template.

Additionally, you could suggest/conduct an audit that isn't already being done and is prompted by awareness of contemporary best practice, new developments or significant events.

Audit can also be used to see whether steps that are taken to improve personal/practice performance have actually been successful. This activity is called 'completing the audit cycle'.

Engages in significant event reviews and learns from them as a team-based exercise.

The second word descriptor in the 'competent' column follows on from our engagement with audit. Similar attitudes and principles apply in that we should recognise that significant events (which are positive as well as negative) are powerful sources of learning, provided they are discussed in suitable settings. Medical communities have mostly moved beyond the culture and expectation of omniscience and the associated reluctance to identify problems or admit errors. Nowadays, significant event reviews are not juries or confessionals, but are meetings in which the complexity of significant events can be understood. Even the most straightforward problem often has structural as well as human dimensions and cumulatively, such events do a great deal to improve patient care (particularly patient safety) and build trust within a team.

A significant event template might contain the following headings:

- **Date** of the event
- **Who the event was discussed with** (e.g. medical colleagues, nurses, team members etc)
- **Description** of the event
- **Issues raised** (consider the issues for yourself, others involved & administrative systems)
- **Learning outcomes**: what went well? What could have been improved upon? Any learning needs identified?
- **Action points**: how were the issues addressed?
- **Changes**: what changes were made? (Consider the issues for yourself, others involved & administrative systems)

Tip: producing evidence of engagement with significant events

The word descriptor is quite specific in that it requires doctors to take part in the process, rather than just understand the theory.

Good evidence would show, preferably from a reflective log such as that shown in the text, that you have picked up on the key points of the discussion, have thought about whether any of these points apply to you and then developed a learning plan related to these.

Even better evidence arises when you bring one of your *own* significant events to be reviewed by the team.

By involving the team and the locality, encourages and facilitates wider participation and application of clinical governance activities

This competency is classed as 'excellent' because having mastered and applied the principles of clinical governance to our own team, we now involve wider groups to improve quality more generally. This degree of expertise requires us to understand the factors that influence quality at locality level and above.

As with several other 'excellent' competencies, we need to show wider awareness of service delivery, the management processes involved and the quality assurance mechanisms that apply. Primary care organisations (PCOs) are relatively strong in dealing with the management and administration aspects of local health care services. However, clinical governance is in comparison, relatively poorly developed in most countries of the UK. This is an area where doctors have a great deal to contribute in that they can comment on the quality markers that might be appropriate to a service. Remember the old adage that **'What is measurable is not always important and what is important is not always measurable'.**

To demonstrate this competency, having understood the wider picture, we can contribute to the data collection required for clinical governance in the locality. More proactively, we might educate the team and other colleagues and encourage them to participate. Beyond this, some doctors advise the PCO on clinical governance, often in relation to areas of special interest in which they have expertise. Many enhanced services have started because of the enthusiasm of local practitioners, who have not only helped to develop the service but also advised on the quality markers that are appropriate. The involvement of clinicians in the development of QOF criteria is another example of this, on a national scale.

What sort of evidence of quality might doctors recommend? Such evidence is of different types and can be used in different ways to support CG. One approach is to think of this evidence as being quantitative or qualitative and as being related to process or outcome. The evidence from QOF can be applied to this framework as shown by Rambihar in the figure below (*Rambihar, B.V. 2005. Defining Evidence of relevance to the Revalidation of General Practitioners that could be developed in Appraisal. University of Dundee. (MMEd-thesis*).

All four quadrants provide valuable material for CG and from the perspective of developing the quality of the service, there is no intrinsic superiority of one type of evidence over another.

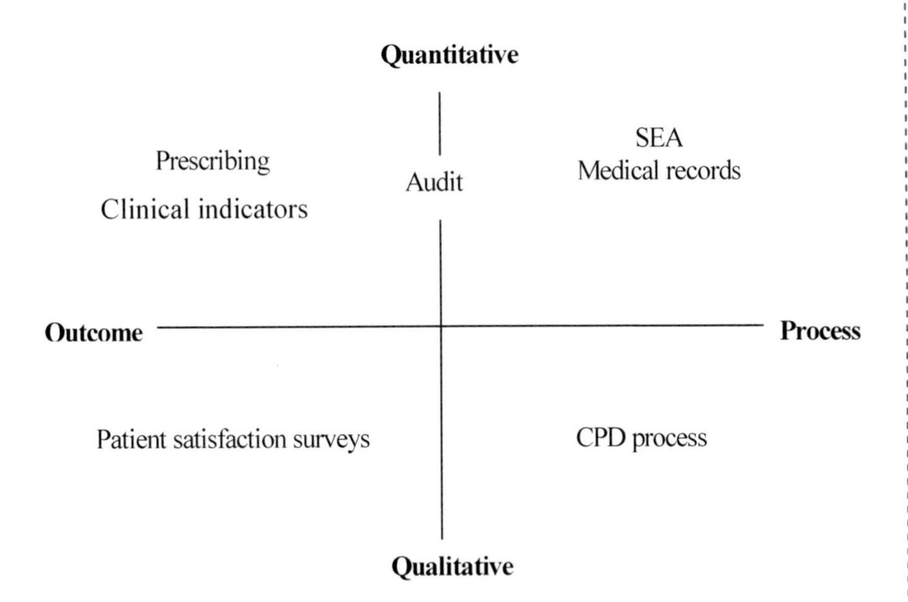

The figure shows how evidence is distributed, but what it does not indicate is that the bulk of the evidence often resides within the upper left quadrant (quantitative outcomes data). These may be regarded by some as 'good' or 'robust' data on the basis that they are numerically measurable and potentially reliable.

However, we should be wary of making such value judgments. Quantitative evidence is valuable but is not necessarily more important than data derived from qualitative sources. Thus SEA may be of more significance in terms of identifying the need for change than statistical data about the service.

Both quantitative and qualitative information should be gained where possible, as the two approaches are complementary in building up a better picture of performance. This principle applies just as much to the performance of *individuals* as it does to the performance of a service.

Tip: developing a wider awareness of clinical governance

PCOs usually have a lead person dealing with clinical governance, who can advise on the locality-wide indices of quality that are used. Most of these are quantitative and are presented as graphs to allow inter-practice comparison.

Look at one of these comparisons and, in discussion with the practice, identify significant differences and suggest why these might be.

What do you think of the indices that are used? Are these relevant/important? Are they measuring simply what *can* be measured, or are they measuring what *should* be?

Is the practice offering any enhanced services on behalf of the locality? If so, look at the contract made with the PCO.

What aspects of the quality of this service are being reported upon? Again, what are your comments on the measures used?

Needs Further Development	Competent for licensing	Excellent
Contributes to the education of students and colleagues.	Identifies learning objectives and uses teaching methods appropriate to these. Assists in making assessments of learners.	Evaluates outcomes of teaching, seeking feedback on performance. Uses formative assessment and constructs educational plans. Ensures students and junior colleagues are appropriately supervised.

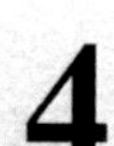

The fourth competency progression takes us into a developing area, that of doctor as teacher. It illustrates how we move from:

Being available and prepared as a non-expert teacher to be involved in the wider educational process

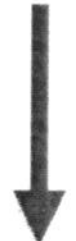

When engaged in teaching, using basic educational principles to teach appropriately and also being prepared (for example by giving feedback) to provide formative assessments of the learner's performance.

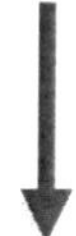

Seeking to improve personal standards of teaching. Becoming more proficient as a teacher by undertaking more structured evaluations and by helping learners to develop educational plans.

Looking at each of the word pictures in turn:

Contributes to the education of students and colleagues.

The first competency is at a basic level and requires us to engage with the education that goes on around us. 'Good medical practice' encourages doctors to regard teaching as being part of routine medical practice. For a non-specialist teacher, this can simply involve playing a role in the educational programs that go on in the practice, for example by allowing students to sit in and observe the consultation, by answering queries of those in training or by becoming more involved in debriefing and case discussion.

The curriculum has a statement devoted to this area, in which it suggests that we should be able to:

- Understand how adults learn
- Demonstrate an awareness of the differing learning styles of individuals
- Demonstrate a learner-centred approach to teaching
- Demonstrate the ability to facilitate the learning of a small group
- Deliver a presentation clearly and effectively, Contribute positively to a culture of teaching and learning within the practice organisation
- Understand the benefits of interprofessional and multiprofessional learning
- Demonstrate the ability to give effective feedback to a colleague

We will consider some of these issues below:

The learners that we come across in general practice are adults, rather than children, and 'adult learning' has some particular characteristics. Being mature and independent individuals, adults particularly value their autonomy and usually, they learn better if allowed to be self-directed. This is not an absolute. For example, it does not mean that learners should be allowed to sink by virtue of having no direction at all. If they are in situations that are entirely new to them, it would be appropriate for the GP to direct their learning rather than leave them to flounder and become dispirited.

Learning through experience is particularly valuable, especially if new experiences are embedded or purposefully connected with previous experiences and insights. In this way, learners can put new knowledge, skills and attitudes into a context that they already understand. Connecting new experiences with old ones is also a mechanism that allows new learning to gain a sense of proportion. We have a role in creating these important connections, for example by asking 'how does this differ from what you already know', 'what would you now do differently?' etc.

The discomfort that learners experience when exposed to situations that they find difficult, is a powerful motivator for learning. Teachers can hopefully 'sensitise' learners so that they learn to recognise their own areas of discomfort and act upon them, rather than ignoring them.

People learn in a variety of ways and no one style is better than another. Doctors can tailor their approach according to what they are trying to achieve and the preferences of the learner. This is explored in the box below:

Main process	Role of teacher
Telling	Passing on knowledge
Questioning	Facilitating learning through awareness-raising questions
Encouraging learning through discovery	Promoting the learner's autonomy and self-directed learning
Exploring feelings and assumptions	Encouraging self-awareness, self-discovery and reflective practice through exploring feelings. Examining assumptions through discussion and judicious challenge

In summary, adult learning is most effective when it is clearly **relevant** to the reality of working life, relates theory to solving **practical** problems and encourages **reflection**. All of these components need to be considered in preparing for teaching.

Learning in primary care is a team exercise. Therefore, learning with other doctors (inter-professional learning) and with other members of the team (multi-professional learning) can be invaluable provided that it addresses shared needs. For example, revising the family planning protocol is better if the doctors and the nurses who run the clinic do so in collaboration.

Teaching is not entirely for the learner's benefit. Indeed, preparation for teaching is an excellent form of continuing professional development because it influences attitudes and behaviour in the consulting room and thereby improves patient care. Educational skill and insight encourages doctors to *see patients as both learners and teachers*, improving shared understanding and therefore the quality of patient management.

Identifies learning objectives and uses teaching methods appropriate to these.

To be 'competent' doctors should demonstrate that they are able to help learners convert broad areas of educational need into manageable tasks or 'objectives '. Objectives should be written in such a way that the task is clear. Good objectives are said to be SMART, meaning that they are:

Specific: clear and concise.
Measurable: written as verbs (e.g. analyse, design, prescribe, inject etc.) rather than as vague objectives (e.g. become aware of, understand, appreciate etc.) which cannot be easily defined or measured.
Achievable: by ensuring that resources (e.g. expertise, time & funding) are available and that the goals are attainable.
Relevant to the aim
Time-bound: with the date for completion being both explicit and realistic.

The teaching methods should address these, but again they need not be complicated. For example, if a learner lacks a skill such as soft tissue injection, s/he may learn better by going to a clinical skills lab or being taught through practical demonstration than by being given a talk or shown a video.

Assists in making assessments of learners.

The second of the 'competent' descriptors refers to our willingness to engage in making formative assessments that assist the learner's development. These assessments need be no more complicated than giving constructive feedback. Many doctors are asked to do this as part of multi-source feedback. Where there is opportunity for the feedback to be more detailed, the principles of doing this effectively should be observed. For example, feedback should be specific, based on evidence such as the observation of behaviour, actionable (i.e. something can be done in relation to it), balanced and feasible.

There are other guidelines about how best to deliver feedback, such as Pendleton's rules, which are worth knowing about.

Evaluates outcomes of teaching, seeking feedback on performance.

Uses formative assessment and constructs educational plans.

Ensures students and junior colleagues are appropriately supervised

These 'excellent' competencies require doctors to show more advanced educational expertise. At present, these abilities may be witnessed in many training practices but doctors who are not involved in education are unlikely to have the need or the opportunity to demonstrate these skills.

In the future, involvement in the teaching of doctors and other primary healthcare professionals will become a more routine part of every GP's core functions at which time, these skills will no longer be the sole concern of specialist educators.

Professionalism

15 Professionalism: Overview of the performance areas

Funny word, 'professionalism'. It sounds very straightforward (we all know what being professional means, don't we?), but arouses strong feelings and passions because many doctors have their own preferred view of what this means. Perhaps that is the heart of it, because professionalism is as much an ideology or creed that we believe in and sign up to as an expectation from profession, society and ourselves of how skilful and effective we should be in our work. Doctors are given a special position of trust in society and professionalism is in large part our way of justifying that privilege. Actually, it's more than that because professionalism is an important way of *creating* trust between patients and ourselves and through this, trust between society and the medical profession.

Why do we need trust? Because being appreciated, even admired, is great but its not enough. Without trust, particularly when the diagnosis or the right way forward is uncertain, as it often is in general practice, we can do much less to help our patients.
Of course, doctors work in teams rather than in isolation and professionalism has a similar role in generating and maintaining trust with colleagues both medical and non-medical.

Professionalism used to be (mainly) defined by the profession, but we are living in an age in which relationships between doctors and their society are maturing. Facilitated by a reduction in the 'power-gap' between the professions and society along with more open dialogue, the nature of professionalism faces challenges and new expectations from a number of directions, especially:

- Less deference to professionals along with increased public accountability
- Increased power and knowledge amongst patients driven by the availability of technical information, more open public debates and the organisation of patients into special interest and lobby groups.
- Increasing diversity of patients particularly in British multicultural society, leading to diversity of expectations.
- The advance of medical technology, with impacts particularly on rationing and medical ethics

We should remember that doctors are not just members of a profession but are part of society. Several of the factors mentioned above will also influence how the doctors of the future wish to see professionalism develop (that means you, by the way!)

What we look for when we assess professionalism?

Trust may be the aim, but it is not a skill we can learn given that it is in the eye of the beholder. Instead, we can develop our professionalism by learning to respect the expectations of profession and society and to show respect to people (including ourselves) and to our professional responsibilities.

The latter are defined by the codes of conduct and laws of profession and society.

Respect is partly an attitude but it is also a number of behaviours that show how 'seriously' (e.g. diligently or thoughtfully) we approach things.

For assessors, a shorthand way of assessing professionalism is to look at the doctor's attitudes and behaviour. Do these indicate that the doctor has, and is able to maintain, the respect that it is required?

Everything in the competence framework seems important but ' professionalism' has a special place. It is the commitment that we make to live our lives in such a way that creates and maintains the trust without which we cannot be good doctors. In short, professionalism underpins everything else that we do and when doctors go seriously wrong, problems with professionalism are often of a large part of the reason.

Professionalism and RDMp

P is manifest through RDM. It is not separate from it. For assessors, this means that when we assess the last two domains, we should look for evidence of professionalism that comes from the first ten.

This means something important for doctors in training. As we showed earlier in the book (see page 9), the three areas of relationship, diagnostics and management (RDM) which in shorthand to describe the first 10 domains, are underpinned by professionalism (P), which is made up of the last two domains. In practical terms, when we say that professionalism underpins RDM, we mean that the competencies described in the last two domains are manifest by the way the doctor demonstrates RD and M.

Let us illustrate this by looking at how professionalism (i.e. **respect** for people, including ourselves and for professional and contractual responsibilities) manifests itself in the other ten domains:

Relationship

This is covered by the competency areas: communicating with patients, practising holistically & working with colleagues and in teams. The underlying theme in these three areas is that of the relationship between doctor and patients/colleagues. To have effective relationships, we show our respect in a number of ways such as:

Communicating well: This means having the respect to be *appropriately attentive*, i.e. showing respect by listening, taking an active interest, trying to understand the viewpoints, concerns and expectations of patients and trying to jointly develop management plans. We also show respect by being *responsive* to patient preferences and modifying plans in the light of discussion. This area describes how professionalism/respect involves exploring and taking account of the patient's values and attitudes, being aware of personal attitudes and taking steps to avoid prejudice. These personal attitudes include being open to the possibility that we might be wrong, for example that we may wrongly class patients as being 'worried well' or 'heartsink' through bias and vulnerabilities of our own.

Practising holistically: showing respect for the patient by being interested enough to explore the impact of the problem on the patient's life. Beyond this, we show professionalism/respect by being interested in the others who are affected by the problem, particularly family members and carers.

Working with colleagues and in teams: professionalism/respect is shown by the way in which we make efforts to establish effective working relationships with people – however different or unfamiliar or difficult the status, personality, style and approach of these people might be. In practical terms we avoid making assumptions about colleagues and make use of their skills appropriately. In addition, by the way in which we seek views, work cooperatively, nurture and reward others in the team. 'Maintaining an ethical approach' describes how professionalism/respect for team members also means providing equality of opportunity, respecting the differences between people (i.e. their diversity) and respecting people enough to want to see them flourish by championing their personal development. More on this later.

Diagnostics

This is covered by the competency areas data gathering, making a diagnosis, clinical management and medical complexity. The underlying theme in these four areas is the process of gathering and interpreting information in order to make justifiable judgements and decisions. Professionalism/respect in this area is shown by:

- Our willingness to involve others (particularly patients) in the decision-making process
- The respect we show to other colleagues involved in patient care though using their skills appropriately and keeping them informed and
- The commitment we show to reach and maintain the decision-making standards of the profession as described in Good Medical Practice

Management

This is covered by the competency areas primary care administration and IMT, community orientation and maintaining performance, learning and teaching. The underlying theme in these three areas is how we deal with the management of the *medical service* that we provide both to individual patients and to the community and with managing our *personal performance*. The main attributes that we require are the abilities to plan, organise, direct and control *people* (including ourselves) and *systems* in order to accomplish a goal. Between them, these are the skills of 'management'.

Primary care administration and IMT: showing professionalism/respect for the patient and the practice by appropriately and diligently using the IT and the protocols that are in place to improve patient care.

Community orientation: showing professionalism/respect for the community by trying to understand the characteristics of the practice population and then tailoring personal actions and the services provided in order to give people what they need (which may not be the same as what they want!). This is also an example of situations in which we show respect for *ourselves* by backing our judgement when we need to.

Maintaining performance, learning and teaching: professionalism/respect for the expectations of the profession and of society is shown by our willingness and capacity to monitor, adapt and improve our own performance. In terms of management, this requires us to have good personal organisational skills so that we can identify and attend to problems and also identify areas of 'weakness' before problems occur in these areas. The latter requires routine monitoring, which in itself depends upon organisation and time management skills.

Poor professionalism as a red flag: Professionalism is widely known to correlate with performance. Good professionalism may predict good performance although the research is not yet clear on this point. At the other end of the spectrum, as the GMC will tell you, doctors who are a cause for significant concern often have problems with their professionalism. If we are assessors, we shouldn't just pass off problems with professionalism as being unfortunate or irritating. The fact that a trainee is often late for work, doesn't make log entries as they should or fails to get immunised may, as individual episodes, be ignored. However, a pattern of such behaviour is significant and should be regarded as a red flag because, as we have seen, poor professionalism undermines most of the behaviours that are required of competent doctors. If picked up early, we may prevent the doctor from failing or (worse) from becoming untrainable.

The deeper features are our DNA. Although few in number, they underpin all the behaviours described in the competence framework and are described in terms of knowledge, skills, attitudes and personal qualities. The behaviours being tested in the 'Professionalism' section are shown in the table below, where the categories indicate the degree of weighting.

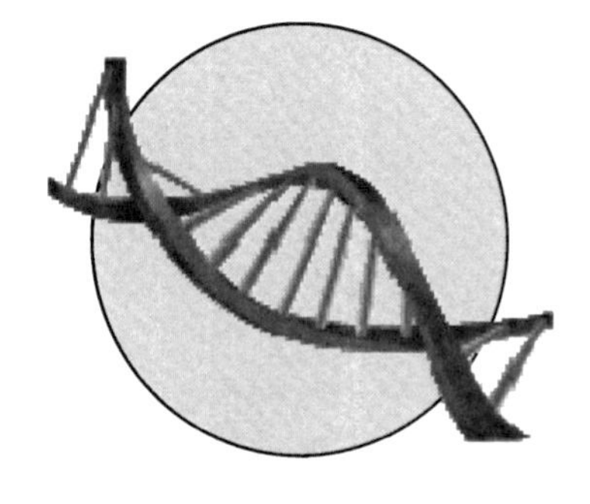

The behaviours are shown in the left-hand column. We will describe these in greater detail to clarify what they are. As you read them, use the table to cross-reference them to the domains that they underpin. This will increase your understanding and help you to develop the skills you need for each area of performance. The weighting will help you here. For example, 'fitness to practise' requires relatively little 'learning & personal development' but relies heavily upon 'coping with pressure'.

If you are (or your trainee is) having a problem with performance in a domain look at the underlying deeper features for guidance on where the problem might lie and therefore which behaviours need working on.

	Maintaining an ethical approach to practice	Fitness to practise
Professional integrity	High	Medium
Learning & personal development		Low
Coping with pressure		High

Professional integrity:

- Respecting and defending the contribution & needs of all. This includes respecting our position as doctors and the special responsibility and protocols of behaviour that this creates. It also includes respecting patients and colleagues.
- Being committed to equality of care for all.
- Treating people fairly with equal concern.
- Discriminating fairly, valuing differences between people and encouraging the development of potential in all.
- Understanding our personal biases and taking these into account when making judgements by ensuring that we do not show unfair bias (positive or negative) toward others.
- Being prepared to justify our decisions, defending these or changing these when appropriate.

Learning & personal development:

- Acknowledging our limitations and identifying what needs to be learned
- Learning both from experience and from targeted study
- Regularly and routinely updating clinical and other job-related skills
- Using the mechanism of personal development to keep up with changes in GP role and skill base

Coping with pressure:

- Being aware of our strengths/limitations. When problem-solving, working within these limits by compromising, delegating and seeking help appropriately
- Remaining calm and under control by using strategies to deal with pressure and stress
- Not losing sight of the wider needs of the situation

What can we learn from the deeper features?

The two competency domains in the 'professionalism' cluster are 'maintaining an ethical approach' and 'fitness to practise'. These complement each other in that the first domain concerns the respect that we show towards *people* whereas the second focuses on the respect we show toward *profession and society*.

'Respect' is an odd word. It doesn't mean that we are passive and deferential. It's an active endeavour that shows a deep-seated commitment on our part to do our best to serve people (including ourselves) with humanity and skill and to live up to what is expected of us.

The deeper features shown above describe many of the important active behaviours that help us to treat people fairly and thereby gain their trust.

Interestingly, as the deeper features show us, the ability to remain fit to practise is strongly associated with the ability to cope with pressure. This means that even if we understand the concept of professionalism and have good ' professional integrity', if we lack the ability to deal with the pressure of patient demands, the competition between work and life, the professional expectations of keeping up-to-date and the challenges of changing role and skill base, then we will have difficulty in maintaining our fitness to practise.

Poor ability to cope is therefore an important indicator that fitness to practise will come under threat if it isn't rectified. During the training period, this may affect progress but in independent life, failure to cope with pressure may lead to serious problems such as performance issues and possibly, GMC involvement.

16 Professionalism: Maintaining an ethical approach to practice

This performance area is about practising ethically with integrity and a respect for diversity.

At first sight, this may seem like a relatively small domain within the competence framework. Don't be fooled! Its ramifications are huge because ethics and its associated values and attitudes underpin virtually every action that a doctor takes. Additionally, these attributes are strongly associated with the trust that patients have in us as individual doctors and with the trust they have in the profession.

To understand these attributes, let's think about how they are used in practice.

Ethics and joint decision-making

Ethics sounds theoretical, but it has real practical significance. One way to consider ethics is to look at its major application in medicine, which is its role in improving decision-making. Remember first of all that in general practice, decision-making is not doctor-centred, but is done in partnership with the patient or the patient's representatives. This decision-making has two major strands. One is the need to practice evidence-based medicine and the other is to accompany this by the use of values-based practice (Fulford KWM. *Ten Principles of Values-Based Medicine.* Ch. 14. In: Radden J (ed.). *The Philosophy of Psychiatry: a companion* New York: Oxford University Press, 2004, pp. 205–34)

The relationship between the two is that Evidence-Based Practice is concerned with complex/conflicting evidence, whereas Values-Based Practice is concerned with complex/conflicting values. Let's pause for a moment to think about this.

Values-based practice

Can you recall any episodes in which complex and conflicting values between yourself and the patient influenced decision-making? When decision-making is difficult, have you ever wondered whether the problem might lie in a difference in values? How would you explore this possibility in consultation? Try it next time things are not going well, perhaps by finding out if there is a mismatch between what the *patient* feels they need and what *you* are hoping to achieve.

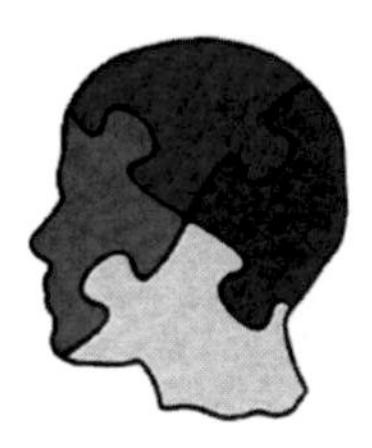

Joined up?
See p14

The rationale for evidence-based medicine is well known but even where the evidence is good, joint decisions should also take into account the values of those involved in the decision. On the doctor's side, values may be informed (even biased) by the views of the team, practice, profession and local health care system and on the patient's side, by the views of family, carers, employers, teachers etc.

So the first step to using ethics in a practical way is to explore and understand our personal values and to do so openly, i.e. without fear of censure. It can sometimes be difficult for educators to provide these opportunities, but doing so is an important way of valuing the diversity of different people's viewpoints.

Is it appropriate to censure the ethics of others? Because people vary so much, there are very few absolutes in ethics and it is through discussion that we learn what is acceptable to the majority and what might not be.

We have to remember that things change. Evidence-based practice changes in response to science and the expectations of society and the profession. It is therefore not a static body of opinion but more a journey than a destination. The same applies to values, particularly in a multicultural society where values are often surprisingly diverse and society's idea of what is acceptable continually changes. This evolution happens best if opportunities for discussion are created without being unfair to those who express views that are 'challenging'. Part of our role as doctors is to encourage society to have these difficult debates. Think, for example, of the prominent role that doctors play in discussions around human fertility and gene therapy. In our professional lifetimes, science is going to make possible what at present seems impossible and as a result, everyone's ethics (profession and society) will be challenged as never before.

Personal values are therefore not fixed in perpetuity and should be informed by a number of people and organisations as discussed above. For the medical profession, the GMC produces 'Good Medical Practice 'which we can think of as a contemporary description of what is acceptable professional behaviour. This is therefore an important document and we should be familiar with it, referring to what it has to say when discussing our performance as practitioners.

In addition, our values will be tempered by knowledge of the legal framework within which we practise. To illustrate this with practical examples, we may apply our values to common situations such as the following:

- Situations where consent and confidentiality are issues, such as treating those with learning disabilities or treating young teenagers.
- Rationing decisions (e.g. doing the greatest good for the greatest number, the implications of implementing guidelines such as NICE, which apply in England but not in Scotland).
- The care of the terminally ill (e.g. euthanasia and advance directives).

Just as our personal values are not set in stone, the views that patients hold will not only change from person to person, but may also change in an individual over time, particularly through the course of a chronic disease or in response to significant life events such as bereavement. For example, someone who may never have thought that suicide was an acceptable option, may find themselves changing their mind when having to endure intolerable suffering.

Beyond understanding our values, we apply ethics to practice through our *reasoning* skills, through gaining *knowledge* of the values likely to be involved in different health care scenarios and through our *communication* skills. The latter are particularly important, because as the competence framework shows us, good communication involves the active use of the patient's values for example in:

- Respecting the patient's agenda and preference for involvement.
- Seeking to understand the patient's context and establishing what is important to them.
- Working in partnership to develop a mutually acceptable plan.

Needs Further Development	Competent for licensing	Excellent
Observes the professional codes of practice, showing awareness of their own values, attitudes and ethics and how these might influence professional behaviour.	Identifies and discusses ethical conflicts in clinical practice.	Anticipates and avoids situations where personal and professional interests might be brought into conflict.

1

This first competency progression is principally about personal values, attitudes and ethical approaches. We move from:

Understanding the basics of Good Medical Practice and discussing how we stand in relation to this.

Correctly identifying situations in which ethical conflicts are an issue and using a framework of ethical principles to clarify our thinking and justify our actions.

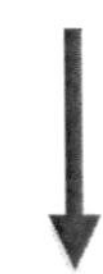

Looking ahead and anticipating potential ethical conflicts, preventing these from occurring wherever possible and being open about conflicts where these are avoidable.

Looking at each of the word pictures in turn:

Observes the professional codes of practice, showing awareness of their own values, attitudes and ethics and how these might influence professional behaviour.

The first step in this progression is for us to recognise that professional codes of practice exist and to try to understand the contents of the GMC document 'Good Medical Practice' (GMP).

Why is this important? A lack of awareness of the broad themes within GMP would be of concern, as this document helps us to gauge, challenge and develop our values.

At this basic level of ability, we may not need to know GMP in detail or be able to skilfully use an ethical framework to argue an ethical problem. However, we should be able to recognise when the problem has attitudinal or ethical dimensions and be able to deduce what these dimensions might be, examples being 'doing the most good' or 'being fair to everyone'. Additionally, we should be able to argue how values, attitudes and ethics, particularly our own, might influence a decision.

The curriculum mentions a number of areas in which personal values may have a bearing on healthcare issues. For example, it states that a doctor should:

- Ensure that personal opinions regarding risk factors for cardiovascular problems (e.g. smoking, obesity, exercise, alcohol, age, race) do not influence management decisions
- Ensure that a patient's weight does not prejudice the information communicated or the doctor's attitude towards the patient.
- Ensure that personal opinion regarding smoking does not influence management decisions for people with respiratory problems.
- Ensure that skin problems are not dismissed as trivial or unimportant by health care professionals.

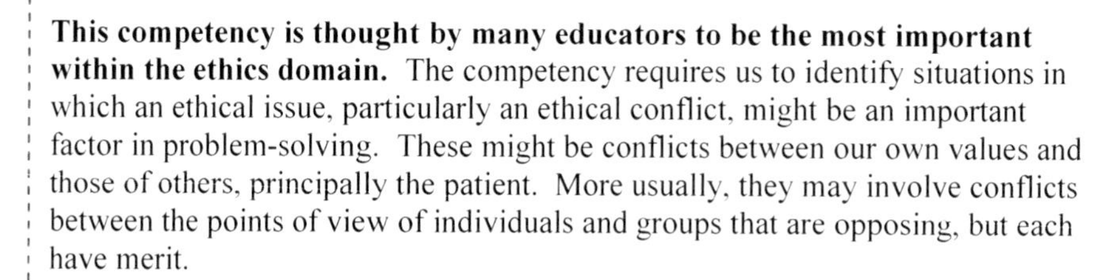

Identifies and discusses ethical conflicts in clinical practice.

This competency is thought by many educators to be the most important within the ethics domain. The competency requires us to identify situations in which an ethical issue, particularly an ethical conflict, might be an important factor in problem-solving. These might be conflicts between our own values and those of others, principally the patient. More usually, they may involve conflicts between the points of view of individuals and groups that are opposing, but each have merit.

An ethical framework, when applied to these areas of conflict, can greatly help to act as a template for discussion, a means of weighing up various aspects of the argument and of justifying whatever decision is finally taken. The ethical framework most commonly used in medicine utilises the following four bioethical principles. This may sound rather dry, but in practice it is an invaluable tool not only for explaining our thoughts and actions to others, but for helping us to clarify our own reasoning.

Autonomy –this concerns respect for individuals and their ability to be self-directed regarding their own health and how they wish to live their lives. Generally, we are expected to recognise, respect and enhance autonomy and actions that diminish autonomy are considered undesirable. As always with ethics, things are not as straightforward as they seem. For example, the rights of the individual have to be balanced with those of society, rationing being a good example. Additionally, there are cultural perspectives with autonomy being much more promoted in the West as a cultural norm than in the East. Neither view is 'right'. Where do *you* stand?

Beneficence - this concept involves making decisions that are best for the patient, without regard to personal gain or the interests of others. No action is wholly good or wholly bad and for GPs, who also have to consider the local community rather than just the individual patient, beneficence is also influenced by utilitarianism, which is the need to ' do the greatest good for the greatest number'.

Non-malificence - means to 'do no harm'. We must refrain from providing ineffective treatments or acting with malice toward patients and this much seems obvious. However, it isn't quite so straightforward because many beneficial therapies also have significant risks. Beneficence therefore has to be balanced with non- malificence and this affects key decisions such as whether to investigate, prescribe, refer or 'watch and wait'. Ultimately it is the patient who

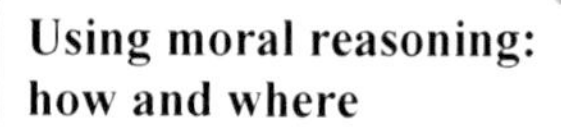

Using moral reasoning: how and where

Values, attitudes and approaches to ethics can be nurtured if we become involved in audit and review meetings, for example when developing practice policies on issues that have ethical implications, such as rationing.

In addition, we often display our understanding of these attributes through case-based discussion and in particular when using 'moral reasoning'.

By this, we mean the ability to problem-solve by applying values and ethics, for example by talking through a case that has an ethical dimension and asking questions about right and wrong, benefit and harm, in relation to those people and groups that might be affected by the decision.
Valuable experience can be gained by attending more formal 'ethics events' such as the local research ethics committee.

Ethical issues are often discussed in the medical press, for example the BMJ publishes the opposing views of two authors on issues that often have ethical underpinnings. In addition, medical matters that have implications for society are discussed in programmes such as the BBC's 'Moral maze'. These are good ways to keep in touch with contemporary thinking.

assigns weight to the risks and benefits through the process of informed decision-making. However, the potential benefits of any intervention must be believed to outweigh the risks in order for the action to be ethical.

Justice means being fair or just to an individual and the wider community in terms of the consequences of an action. Two notions are encapsulated by this term. The first is equality or '*distributive* justice' which is the principle of treating everyone equally. The second is fairness or '*procedural* justice', which means ensuring that the process of making decisions is fair and that undue bias or prejudice is avoided.

Confidentiality is mentioned here because although it is not a single ethical principle in itself, it is a mixture of several of the ethical principles mentioned above. Confidentiality is a very frequent concern of doctors (see box on this page).

As well as understanding the ethical principles that underpin behaviour, we need to observe the laws of the land, some of which compel us to act in particular ways. For example, in England and Wales confidential information must be shared under particular circumstances such as:

- The notification of births and deaths
- Communicable disease
- Abortion
- Serious accidents covered under the Health and Safety at Work
- Prevention of Terrorism Act

These situations may not seem to be contentious, but as health professionals we sometimes need to question the law on behalf of our patients. Complying with the law should therefore never be a substitute for using moral reasoning.

Finally, here are a few examples from the curriculum that demonstrate the wide range of topics that have ethical implications:

- Be able to balance the autonomy of patients who have visual problems with public safety
- Ensure that the risks of diabetic complications are not over-stated in order to coerce a patient into complying with treatment.
- Describe the ethical principles involved when treating an incompetent patient (e.g. unconscious), and when treating a patient who is unable to communicate (e.g. dysphasic).
- Describe the ethical aspects of managing patients/families with genetic conditions, being aware of the issues involved in genetic testing, such as confidentiality, testing children, and pre-symptomatic testing.
- Be able to identify ethical aspects of clinical practice relating to IM&T e.g. security, confidentiality, use of information for insurance company use etc.

Have you come across these situations? Can you think of examples of your own?

Discussion point: examples of areas of ethical conflict involving confidentiality

Where a doctor has concerns over a patient's fitness to drive, for example an epileptic who is not taking their medication and is posing a risk to the public.

Where a patient threatens serious harm to another individual.

Where a doctor believes a patient to be the victim of abuse and the patient is unable to give or to withhold consent to take this further, for example through immaturity or diminished mental incapacity.

Where a doctor has a patient who is a health professional and has concerns that this person is unfit to practice.

Anticipates and avoids situations where personal and professional interests might be brought into conflict.

At the 'excellent' end of this progression, we are able to show insight and honesty even in the face of temptation to do otherwise. The reason for raising conflict of interest as an issue is that trust between doctors and patients and doctors and colleagues may be damaged by situations in which financial or other personal interests affect, or could be feared to affect, professional judgment.

All doctors will be familiar with the situation where drug companies offer gifts, meals etc. in order to literally 'curry favour' and thereby influence future decision-making. We might think that we are beyond such influence and if we do, we should ask ourselves 'Why do commercially astute companies still continue to use these mechanisms?'

As doctors become more senior, the opportunities for temptation increase, for example chances arise to travel to meetings abroad, give presentations and so on. Especially when couched as 'education' it can be hard to see where the conflict lies, but with writing and presentation, competing interests should be made explicit so that colleagues can decide for themselves whether what is being presented might be influenced by payments, sponsorship or other benefits.

Potential conflicts may also arise with financial dealings, for example when a commercial service is also being offered to patients. Doctors who have a commercial stake in nursing homes or pharmacies used by their patients may find themselves in this situation. Likewise, doctors may have a stake in providing private services such as health checks and should take care not 'recommend' them to their patients. To keep actions above board, the doctor may wish to note on the patient's record when an unavoidable conflict of interest arises.

Gifts are a common (although relatively pleasant?) ethical challenge and it would be easy to fool ourselves that the patient is simply being given the opportunity to express thanks. However, gifts may be misinterpreted as a form of payment or inducement and we can prevent conflict arising by not encouraging patients to give, lend or bequeath money or gifts that will directly or indirectly benefit us. The way in which gifts are managed is a good example of the practice's ethical approach, so for example gifts such as donations may be pooled in a practice fund rather than be kept by an individual.

Conflict may also occur at the personal level. For example, it can be difficult to act as a doctor for someone who is also a working colleague such as a partner in practice. Confidentiality will be a constant challenge and dilemmas may occur when medical advice such as a recommendation to take time off sick is in conflict with the interests of the practice.

As we can see, good doctors behave ethically and are seen to be doing so. At this level of performance, doctors will anticipate where problems might arise and discuss with colleagues, take advice (e.g. from a professional or a defence body) and make conflicts clear to others where these are genuinely unavoidable. 'Anticipation' also means using insight to identify a potential problem where this has not previously been recognised. By acting in this way we not only help ourselves, but improve medical care more widely.

Debating points

Although current 'politically correct' thinking dictates that the doctor and patient are partners in diagnosis and treatment, in reality the patient is very dependent and vulnerable.

How does this affect the doctor's wish to promote autonomy?

Should patients who have knowingly contributed to their ill-health be allowed the same access, free of conditions, to NHS services as those who have not?

Ethical approaches

How does your practice deal with gifts from patients? What is your opinion of the approach? Have they identified other areas of ethical conflict for which a joint approach has been developed?

Can you think of any area that should be considered and if so, what would protocol would you devise for the practice on the issue?

Assessor's corner: anticipating ethical conflicts

'Anticipation' is a mechanism by which ethical insight and motivation come together to prevent adverse 'ethical events'. Where does this happen in your practice? Who have you observed doing it? How often have *you* raised an ethical issue?

Ethics is intended to help us make better decisions. As many significant decisions are made in practice meetings, how often is an ethical angle introduced to help problem-solving in these meetings?

Needs Further Development	Competent for licensing	Excellent
Treats patients, colleagues and others equitably and with respect for their beliefs, preferences, dignity and rights.	Recognises and takes action to address prejudice, oppression and unfair discrimination within the self, other individuals and within systems.	Actively promotes equality of opportunity for patients to access health care and for individuals to achieve their potential.

2

The second competency progression concerns our respect for others and our views on fairness, which includes equity, equality of opportunity and access. We move from:

Respecting others and treating them with fairness

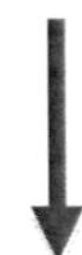

Being open and honest about our own prejudice and unfair bias and looking to minimise these in ourselves and our organisation

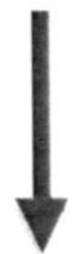

Influencing the ethos of the organisation so that practical steps are taken to improve equality of opportunity in personal development and service provision.

Looking at each of the word pictures in turn:

Treats patients, colleagues and others equitably and with respect for their beliefs, preferences, dignity and rights.

This competency progression puts an emphasis on *equality* whereas the next concerns *diversity*. The two are related in that they both require us to show appropriate respect toward others and to treat people with fairness. This can't happen without self-awareness coupled with awareness of the life experience, power and degree of control that other people have.

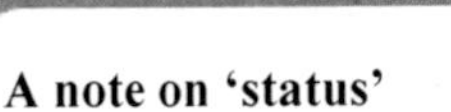

A note on 'status'

There is difference between being seen to be understanding and fair and being perceived as a little 'superior' and the difference lies much more in attitude than appearance.

Although status can be a privilege for those who work in the professions, for doctors it can sometimes be an impediment in relating to patients, which we need to be aware of and manage.

In this progression, the basic level of performance is to show the fairness and respect that every good citizen would expect to show, and be shown, in British society. You may think that this is easy to do. However, it may be harder for doctors to do than the 'average' citizen because doctors have power and privilege that can act a barrier to understanding the powerlessness and inequity that others in society feel. As a result it can be difficult to appreciate how this gap can lead to fewer options and poorer medical care.

Assessor's corner:treating people with respect

Showing respect is a persistent and consistent behaviour applied to various types of people and personalities.

Good evidence comes from patient and colleague feedback. However, asking about and taking account of the preferences of patients and colleagues is an important early stage of showing respect.

As educators we should listen out for and nurture curiosity and interest of this type. Although respect should be felt in the heart, it can be developed from the head.

Therefore, doctors who have the curiosity to ask about what others are thinking are already developing the mindset of respect.

The importance of self-awareness was mentioned above and the curriculum gives us some examples of topic areas in which awareness is particularly important. The doctor should:

- Have a balanced view of benefits and harms of medical treatment
- Discuss their own values, attitudes and approach to ethical issues (e.g. termination of pregnancy, contraception for minors, consent, confidentiality, cosmetic surgery)
- Ensure that their own beliefs, moral or religious reservations about any contraceptive methods or abortion do not adversely affect the management of a patient's sexual health.
- Understand that their own attitudes and feelings are important determinants of how they manage:
    - ⇒ people who self harm
    - ⇒ people who misuse drugs or alcohol
    - ⇒ people who know more about their illnesses than their doctors do
    - ⇒ people who for many reasons engender strong emotions in us.
- Understand the importance of issues for the doctor such as their family of origin and personal prejudices.

Respecting other people's preferences, dignity and rights requires us to show an interest in patients' thoughts and try to accommodate these as far as we can. It's easy to hide behind our professional position and not actually go very far; tokenism is pretty widespread. Try asking: suppose you were a doctor who believed in patients as partners, rather than just believing that this was a politically correct slogan that had little importance. How much further would you go in accommodating patients' preferences?

Respect is therefore not a passive act but requires interest, communication and good negotiation both to elicit preferences and to negotiate their place in a management plan. Preferences arise from a number of sources including personal, societal and cultural factors and can cause conflict when they leads to risk, conflict or both. For instance, a patient may refuse an intimate examination where this has been recommended and this will raise an ethical dilemma and possibly, depending on the perceived risk, conflict between the patient and their doctor or their family.

Recognises and takes action to address prejudice, oppression and unfair discrimination within the self, other individuals and within systems.

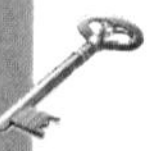

<u>Being fair</u>

Many educators regard this as being one of the most important competencies in this area. To demonstrate this competence, we move from simply giving respect to recognising the threats to fairness and respect that might occur, and then preventing these from taking place or from having a deleterious influence.

This complex competency is the bedrock of becoming, and continuing to be, a fair person as well as a fair doctor. The wording 'prejudice, oppression and unfair discrimination' may be off-putting. For example, although many of us would admit to the possibility of being prejudiced, how many of us recognize ourselves as being capable of oppression or unfair discrimination? Although these attributes may not be visible at work, perhaps they show themselves in our private lives? Ask your partner or family! If it is genuine, the ability to be fair should apply as much to our lives outside patient care as within it.

Beyond observing the laws and codes of practice as described earlier, we need self-awareness, openness and the opportunity to talk in a protected environment about our personal feelings and experiences of 'prejudice, oppression and unfair discrimination'. The minute we begin to open up about these issues from a personal viewpoint we are already en route to becoming a fairer practitioner. It would be impossible (and inappropriate) to attempt to bring our personal biases into line with our peers, as these biases are important sources of our diversity. Diversity as we will soon discuss, is valuable and necessary to teams and to society. However, we need to identify, explore and understand our personal set of values, biases and prejudices so that these can be taken into account when making judgements. This applies especially to prejudices, which are biases that have no basis in reason or legitimacy but are nevertheless ubiquitous.

Dealing with personal issues is not a 'once and for all' event as prejudice changes with, for example, the expectations of society and personal experience. It needs to be kept under review so that we don't simply become more inflexible or intolerant as we become more experienced. Dialogue is important because what is 'fair' is partly governed by the views of society as well as our own ethical principles.

We cannot maintain fairness simply through self-reflection. Discussion is also important partly because this is how we get the feedback that keeps our excesses in check. Additionally, we have to feel okay about ourselves before commenting on other people and discussion with people we respect is a good way of achieving this.

This competence describes three levels (self, other individuals, systems) but these are not the elements of a hierarchy. Without self-awareness and personal action, what we have to say about the other levels may lack insight, conviction and validity. It is neither necessary nor possible to be blameless in order to comment on others. Nevertheless, we should be humble enough to recognise the weaknesses of our own position when making such comments.

It may seem presumptuous to comment on other people, but it is a facet of positions of authority and leadership. For doctors, there is a need to do so because of our role in delivering a service whose quality depends on the performance of many individuals and systems. Although we may think of ourselves as being independent practitioners, in reality we are inter-dependent.

Constructive comments with the aim of keeping the system fair for those who work within it and for the patients we work for, are therefore necessary. However, taken beyond a certain point this can become oppression, which is unacceptable. The dividing line is not static and to be competent, we need to know what to look for that may alert us that the dividing line is being crossed.

Discrimination

Discrimination is the ability to separate people or items on the basis of some marker of quality. We shouldn't be afraid of being discriminating because it is a necessary part of making judgements. Of course, a balance is needed and the important thing is to ensure that discrimination remains fair. We should not be so undiscriminating that *no* judgement is made, nor so unfairly discriminating (which means positively as well as negatively) that our judgments may not be sound. Discrimination is therefore not only appropriate, but also vital both in clinical practice and in dealing with colleagues and employees.

Equal opportunities

Doctors also select people to positions of responsibility, which may range from opportunities to lead a particular task to being formally employed. A condition,

How important is 'acting fairly' to you?

How do we feel about fairness? Is it important but not central to our lives, or is it part of our integrity as human beings? Remember that integrity is that sense of being 'whole' that we protect from being violated.

Ask yourself whether you feel that fairness is part of your integrity and whether it is something that you would protect in a situation where it was under threat. Such threats are commonplace.

It is all too easy to treat people less well because they are older, junior in hierarchy, because we don't warm to them, because we are stressed or tired and so on. When do you behave less fairly than you should?? How can you prevent this?

Assessor's corner: is the doctor becoming oppressive and unfair?

There are a number of ways of looking at this, for example, how authoritarian is the doctor as a team member? How rigid are his/her views and how does the doctor deal with pressure points e.g. seeing patients who come late/DNA/ ask for emergency or late visits?

What does MSF/informal feedback/SEA say about the doctor's attitudes and actions?

Looking at this from another angle, does the doctor show the ability to detect prejudice and oppression in others? How good is their judgement on these matters? Would they act appropriately and sensitively?

Insights into performance might be gained through actual or hypothetical examples and scenarios.

requirement, or practice that has the effect of unjustifiably excluding or having an adverse impact on a group is covered by equal opportunities legislation that helps to guide the appropriate mindset, for example:

- The Race Relations Act
- The Sexual Discrimination
- The Disability Discrimination Act
- The Employment Equality (Age, Sexual Orientation Religion or Belief) Regulations

What are the key 'people' factors that are subject to unfair discrimination?

Gender
Race
Colour
Nationality
Ethnic or National Origin
Religion or Religious Belief
Disability
Sexuality ('Sexual orientation')
Transgender
Age

Taking action

Doctors may witness prejudice etc. in colleagues and systems and discuss these with those involved. To demonstrate competence, doctors need to know how to recognise prejudice, oppression and unfair discrimination, be vigilant for the signs of these and raise concerns appropriately and sensitively when they occur or discuss how they might do so.

The risks are high, because no person and indeed no organisation, likes to imagine that they have been unfair. Therefore, doctors should seek out the facts, clarify misunderstandings, take advice from colleagues and only then take personal action. This sequence reflects how doctors might address performance issues more broadly and this is discussed in greater detail in the next chapter.

On the equal opportunities front, there are a number of positive actions that can be taken such as:

- Having targets and quotas for disadvantaged and under-represented groups (positive discrimination).
- Monitoring to make sure that unfair discrimination is not taking place, for example with appointments to new posts.
- Looking for and acting on harassment and victimization.
- Having a genuine occupational qualification requirement when making appointments, rather than some spurious one that may indirectly discriminate.
- Monitoring.
- Offering flexible working for employees and flexible service provision for patients.

Unfair positive discrimination

We all have 'forceful features' which can subconsciously (and therefore without our awareness) influence our opinion in a positive or negative direction. For example on the positive side, we can be drawn towards people who are physically attractive or well spoken and also toward people who are like ourselves or remind us of someone we feel positively toward etc. Can you think of any such examples? What are your own forceful features? In which situations would you try to raise your awareness of them? How?

Actively promotes equality of opportunity for patients to access health care and for individuals to achieve their potential.

At the 'excellent' end of the competency progression, we apply our understanding of fairness and equality more widely. 'Equality' is partly to do with the ethical principle of equity and fairness for all. It also overlaps with the law about equal opportunities as discussed earlier. Through personal example and discussion, we can help others including the organisation to understand the importance of these principles and to incorporate them as part of our core values.

What action might we take? We might, for example identify the issue of opportunity and fairness as it relates to management and leadership in primary health care e.g.

- The approaches to the use of resources / rationing.
- Approaches to involving the public and patients in decision-making.
- Appointments to a post or task.
- Patient services and whether a new service might be unfair to some in terms of availability and accessibility.
- Rules governing the access to services. For example, mandatory weight loss or smoking cessation prior to NHS surgery.

The curriculum has some examples that relate to equality of opportunity in patient care. It suggests:

- Ensure that a patient's hearing impairment or deafness does not prejudice the information communicated or doctor's attitude towards the patient.
- Recognise that male circumcision is important for several religious groups.
- All citizens should have equal rights to health and equitable access to health and health information according to their needs.
- Integration is not simply a matter of acquiring skills but of showing commitment. Inclusion begins with commitment to the development of fully accessible services.
- Patients with learning difficulties are more prone to the effects of prejudice and unfair discrimination and doctor's have a duty to recognise this within themselves, other individuals and within systems and to take remedial action.

The underlying principle at work in this competency is that we promote equality of opportunity in the development of team members and, for patients, equality of opportunity to access services.

We also have a role as leaders, which is why the competency refers to the doctor not just providing opportunities, but also actively trying to help individuals to 'achieve their potential'.

Assessor's corner: is the doctor discriminating and doing so fairly?

Does the doctor discriminate between different levels of quality e.g. in their own work or regarding the performance of others?

Is the basis of this discrimination fair, or are irrelevant or unjustified factors brought in? Does the justification lack insight?

Look at the degree of insight that the doctor shows when discussing the ratings that are given by assessors and by *themselves* to structured assessments, especially CbD and COT.

This mindset transposes to patient care in that the best doctors don't just deal with current problems, but try to encourage patients to improve i.e. to achieve *their* potential of being healthy in physical and psychological terms.

Assessor's corner: is the doctor addressing prejudice?

To address the issues, the doctor must first recognize them. Evidence may come through events or through the discussion of hypothetical cases.

Does the doctor admit to having prejudices? (we all have them!). What changes has s/he made or proposed?

Where the doctor recognizes a personal issue, evidence of appropriate action to address prejudice etc. may come through the learning cycle, i.e. raising aspects of personal behaviour as issues for discussion with clinical/non-clinical colleagues and then taking steps to identify needs and attend to them.

Needs Further Development	Competent for licensing	Excellent	
Recognises that people are different and does not discriminate against them because of those differences.	Recognises and takes action to address prejudice, oppression and unfair discrimination within the self, other individuals and within systems.	Values diversity by harnessing differences between people for the benefit of practice and patients alike.	**3**

The third competency progression builds on the previous one by considering the challenges and benefits of diversity. We move from:

Recognizing the ways in which people are different from each other and avoiding personal prejudice related to this.

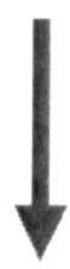

Having identified prejudice within ourselves or within others, taking appropriate action to address the issue.

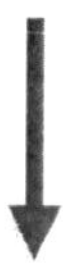

Valuing diversity by understanding the practical uses to which it can be put and being instrumental in doing so.

Looking at each of the word pictures in turn:

Recognises that people are different and does not discriminate against them because of those differences.

Diversity, meaning the differences between people is valuable, but because it is often misunderstood it is insufficiently applied. A radio broadcaster exhorted us by saying 'We are given diversity; let us not turn this into division.'

When diversity is appropriately used, it:

- Builds on the mindset of promoting equality and avoiding unfair bias and prejudice
- Assumes pluralism, which is the belief that the numerous distinct ethnic, religious, or cultural groups present in society are desirable and socially beneficial. On this basis, diversity is pro-active
- Is proactive, recognizing talent, celebrating and harnessing individual differences
- Is inclusive and internally initiated
- Means each person is treated and valued as unique; including background, heritage, economic class, personality and experience

Assessor's corner: 'taking action to promote equality and access'

How well does the doctor feel that equality fairness and respect are shown within the practice? What suggestions does s/he have to improve matters?

What subject area could the doctor audit to investigate a discrimination issue? For example modification of call systems for the deaf, disabled access to the surgery and service access for commuters.

Do the membership of the team and the way the service is provided suggest that equal opportunity is being practised?

What does the doctor think about: the practice development plan, how much personal development is promoted within the team, how accessible training courses are, staff turnover? What does MSF say about the doctor?

What is diversity?

If diversity means differences between people, then the differences that we can define include gender, sexuality, disability, ethnicity, religion and social class. As we can see, the range of differences is broad but discussions on diversity often get no further than discussions about cultural differences. For us to achieve this baseline competency, we need to understand diversity more broadly. In addition, we need to understand diversity in terms of its *purpose* rather than just its knowledge base.

To expand on this, we often get bogged down by learning about *factual* differences between cultural groups. This is not a useful approach because unlike scientific subjects, say biochemistry, diversity is not entirely knowable. That is not to say that knowledge is useless. For example, it can be helpful to know what, in broad terms, the health beliefs and expectations of different ethnic groups might be. However, even these 'facts' are not stable but change in relation to factors such as the process of acclimatisation to a new culture and changes in society itself.

Try thinking of diversity *not as a subject, but as an attitude*. Doctors who really understand diversity show sensibility and cultural humility toward people, rather than just a knowledge of facts. Why humility? Because they do not presume to know the patient's thoughts and do not make assumptions that people, by virtue of their background, will behave or think in particular ways. Instead of treating people as stereotypes (which is so easily done), they encourage people to talk about their perspective and then seek to learn from this.

Empowering people to communicate is important because those who are culturally or socially different often feel reticent to communicate their views for fear of being ridiculed or misunderstood.

Valuing diversity is therefore of practical use, in helping us to feel confident and competent in dealing with people from different backgrounds, different sociological groups and different cultures. We need to remember that 'people' includes our colleagues as well as our patients.

How to understand diversity

Understanding diversity means understanding and *valuing* the differences between people. To do this, we first need to know what those differences are and then judge, in our terms as well as in terms of the other person, what value these differences bring. We shouldn't assume that differences are *always* valuable, but at least we should be open to the possibility.

A parallel example is with team development, where experience teaches us that functional teams are diverse in that they comprise a *variety* of personalities rather than being made up of just one personality type. Therefore, a team might have someone who is good on the theoretical aspects of a problem and another who hates the theory but likes the practicalities of putting things into action. Both are needed

Assessor's corner: does the doctor understand the value of diversity?

What does the doctor value about people who are different or about ideas that are different from his/her own?

Try suggesting examples and evaluating the response. Which types of people/ positions/values does the doctor find particularly *hard* to value? Is this appropriate or does the doctor have a point?

if the team is to work well.

Theorists help to justify what the team seeks to do, but without completer-finishers nothing ever gets done! These different types may in personal terms initially find it difficult to get on, but are likely to do so when they value what the other can do.

Likewise with diversity, a group of people who have different perspectives can greatly enhance joint endeavours. How does this help us in practice life? One significant example is that understanding and valuing a different perspective from our own can improve shared decision-making both in the consultation with patients and with colleagues.

To understand differences we need to continually explore and compare the viewpoints and values of others with our own attitudes and dispositions. This is a lifelong process of discovery, which will not be entirely joyous as there will be frequent challenges to our mindset and periodic conflict between different perspectives and values.

As the word picture indicates, to demonstrate this competency we have to show that we understand diversity. In terms of behaviour, we may not be able to apply our understanding of diversity to practice, but our behaviour should show that we do not discriminate against people because of, for example, cultural or social differences.

Recognises and takes action to address prejudice, oppression and unfair discrimination within the self, other individuals and within systems.

This competency is common to equality and fairness (as discussed in the previous competency progression) and to diversity. It has been covered in depth on page 190. In addition to what has already been said, we should look at our own behaviour and at the behaviour of those we work with and address prejudice that is based on differences.

Values diversity by harnessing differences between people for the benefit of practice and patients alike.

Remember that differences do not just relate to the obvious, such as racial prejudice, but to factors that are more subtle. For example, we may be intolerant of people who have different upbringings such as different schooling (e.g. private versus state sector), have different political or cultural values, who dress differently or are difficult to understand because of language or accent. Prejudice, which may simply start with irritation, seriously impairs our willingness to recognize and learn from what others have to contribute.

The approach taken to achieving this competency is similar to the approach described for 'actively promoting equality of opportunity' (see page 193) . In addition to promoting an appropriate culture within the organization, we need to understand how diversity can be applied to useful effect. Making use of diversity is not a matter of being politically correct. It should be done because it is *useful* to do so.

A group with diverse perspectives better reflects the multicultural nature of British society and will be more representative of what society needs and wants.

What does 'harnessing differences' mean? Sometimes, diversity can be harnessed in relation to a specific problem. For example, a sizeable ethnic minority community may need targeted attention from healthcare workers with a particular understanding of the needs and concerns of that community. Remember that diversity is not just about differences in culture. For instance, the diverse perspectives of the patient population could be used to advise on practice development. However, how prevalent is this? For example, how many practices discuss the development of an adolescent health clinic with teenagers in the community?

In our leadership role, we can demonstrate this competency by being proactive in seeking out talent and in putting people together who are different, but potentially complementary. Of course, differences can be irritating or even frightening and we should not assume that such people will automatically communicate well or get on. If diversity is to be made use of, the problems as well as the potential must be recognized and discussed so that individuals can work fruitfully together.

If diversity is already understood by the organisation, we may wish to perform a diversity audit looking at such criteria as: are opportunities being given so that the talent within the team is recognized and rewarded? Does the profile of people in positions of responsibility reflect the diversity of the team? If not, why might this be and what action needs to be taken?

In the end, equality and diversity are steppingstones to seeing people as individuals rather than as categories or stereotypes. No-one wants to be selected because of the requirement for organisations to comply with 'equal opportunities' or with 'diversity awareness'. People need to be understood, valued and promoted on the basis of who they are as individuals and what they have to offer. The attention given to equality and diversity reflects the fact that misunderstanding and prejudice are widespread and need to be overcome. British society has moved a great deal in recent years in the direction of valuing its multiculturalism and the example that doctors set as role models is as important to society as it is to the profession.

17 Professionalism: Fitness to practise

This competency area is about the doctor's awareness of when his/her own performance, conduct or health, or that of others might put patients at risk and the action taken to protect patients.

The document 'Good Medical Practice' is the key. This area of the competence framework is in large part informed by how the profession itself defines professionalism through this document. GMP is written in generic terms for all medical specialties and then fleshed out in more detail within the context of each specialty. 'GMP for GPs' is therefore an important resource document for us as generalists. Through its descriptions of the unacceptable and the exemplary GP, it helps us understand the standards that we must abide by in professional life and also helps us to benchmark our own performance in relation to these standards.

There are five themes in the performance area 'Fitness to practise'. The first three concern the **maintenance of optimal performance** in the following areas:

- professional performance
- work-life balance
- health

The fourth and fifth themes deal with how we engage in **specific feedback loops** i.e.

- monitoring ones own performance & that of colleagues
- responding to feedback (in particular, complaints)

These are elaborated through the competency progressions, which we will now consider in more detail.

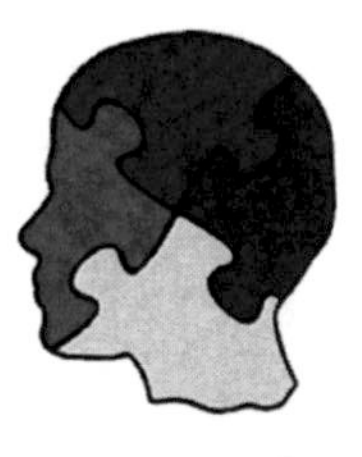

Joined up?
See p14

Needs Further Development	Competent for licensing	Excellent
Understands and maintains awareness of the GMC duties of a doctor.	Observes the accepted codes of practice in order to minimise the risk of disciplinary action or litigation.	Encourages scrutiny and justifies professional behaviour to colleagues.

1

This first competency progression is principally about understanding our professional duties as set out in key documents such as Good Medical Practice and showing the ability to monitor and justify our own performance. We move from:

Understanding our duties as described by the broad themes of GMP.

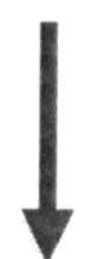

Monitoring our performance and comparing personal standards with the expectations of the profession, for example by using GMP as a tool rather than simply a reference document.

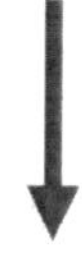

Participating proactively in the process of performance review and clinical governance, for example by using audit or by encouraging feedback on consultations.

Looking at each of the word pictures in turn:

Understands and maintains awareness of the GMC duties of a doctor.

To achieve this competency, we must demonstrate that we understand these duties, by being familiar with GMP. At the competent level (the next step up) we would also need to demonstrate that we can *apply* this understanding to practise.

To understand GMP, we need to know its range and the standards so we will begin with a brief summary of GMP and then consider the situations in which GMP is seriously breached to the extent that the GMC might be involved. This sounds rather dramatic, but understanding the latter helps us to ensure that our standards are kept well within these limits.

Overview of GMP

In broad terms, the GMC requires GPs to provide care that is 'effective, personal and safe'. To continue in independent practice, we have to demonstrate through revalidation that our conduct justifies the trust that is placed in us by patients.

GMP sets out the standards of competence, care and conduct expected of us, under the following main headings:

Good clinical care –to provide good standards of clinical care within the limits of our competence, ensuring that patients are not put at unnecessary risk.
Maintaining good medical practice –to keep up to date with developments in general practice, maintaining our skills and auditing our performance.
Relationships with patients– to develop and maintain successful relationships with our patients.
Working with colleagues – to work effectively with our colleagues.
Teaching and Training– where we have teaching responsibilities, to develop the skills, attitudes and practices of a competent teacher.
Probity –to be honest and trustworthy.
Health – to ensure that any problem with our health does not endanger patients.

We can become more familiar with these by dividing them under the GMC's four performance areas. These are the performance areas that are used in annual GP appraisal:

Knowledge, skills and performance
Maintain professional performance
Apply knowledge and experience to practice
Keep clear, accurate and legible records

Safety and Quality
Put into effect systems to protect patients and improve care
Respond to risks to safety
Protect patients from any risk posed by the doctor's health

Communication, partnership and team work
Communicate effectively
Work constructively with colleagues and delegate effectively
Establish and maintain partnerships with patients

Maintaining Trust
Show respect for patients
Treat patients and colleagues fairly and without prejudice
Act with honesty and integrity

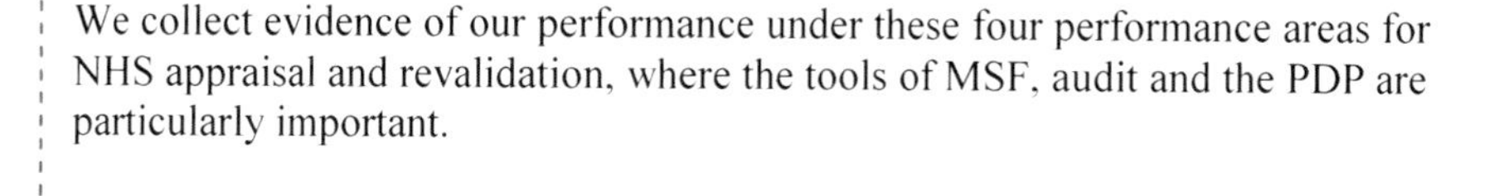

We collect evidence of our performance under these four performance areas for NHS appraisal and revalidation, where the tools of MSF, audit and the PDP are particularly important.

Assessor's corner: is the doctor is aware of GMP?

Evidence may come from professional conversations, e.g. in teaching sessions or through case-based discussion. For example, does the doctor know and understand the GMP headings?

A good test of this is to ask what evidence the doctor would collect under each heading and to ask which GMP headings would be covered by a particular piece of evidence (e.g. the PDP)

With reference to these headings, what behaviours would suggest that a doctor might be underperforming or even be a cause for concern?

Serious breaches of GMP

Most doctors achieve the high standards of GMP, but the GMC has legal powers to take action in the small number of cases where 'Serious or persistent failures to meet the standards puts registration at risk'.

The GMC reassuringly recognise that: 'All human beings make mistakes' Whilst one-off mistakes need to be investigated by those immediately involved, harm addressed and lessons learned, they are unlikely in themselves to indicate a fitness to practise problem. So what constitutes such a problem?

A question of fitness to practise is likely to arise if:

A doctor's performance has harmed patients or put patients at risk of harm
For example, if a series of incidents cause concern. These incidents may indicate persistent technical failings or other repeated departures from good practice which are not being, or cannot be, safely managed locally.

A doctor has shown a deliberate or reckless disregard of clinical responsibilities towards patients
An isolated lapse from high standards of conduct – such as an atypical rude outburst– would not in itself suggest a fitness to practise issue. But the sort of misconduct, whether criminal or not, which indicates a lack of integrity on our part, an unwillingness to practise ethically or responsibly or a serious lack of insight into clear examples of poor practice could bring our registration into question.

A doctor's health is compromising patient safety

A doctor has abused a patient's trust or violated a patient's autonomy or other fundamental rights.
This is a situation in which we act without regard for the patient's rights or feelings, or we abuse our professional position.

A doctor has behaved dishonestly, fraudulently or in a way designed to mislead or harm others
In this situation, our behaviour is such that public confidence might be undermined if the GMC does not take action.

Observes the accepted codes of practice in order to minimise the risk of disciplinary action or litigation.

As we have seen above, to achieve the competent level of performance we must understand GMP and the circumstances in which it is seriously breached. However, the intention is not simply to avoid disciplinary action and litigation, but to maintain and improve standards in line with personal, professional and patient expectations.

The standards that are expected relate mainly to clinical performance but also cover personal health, ethical views and trustworthiness including honesty. Ethics and conflict of interest are covered in the chapter 'maintaining an ethical approach' and in the current chapter we will look more closely at maintaining performance and personal health.

Professional performance

The Chief Medical Officer in his paper on 'Revalidation principles' has stated that the approach to maintaining standards will be to encourage doctors to 'keep up to date and improve their practice, through continuous professional development and reflective practice'. The paper goes on to state that the information on performance available to individuals through clinical governance will be made more available, so that judgements can be better informed.

This approach is already incorporated in WPBA. Essentially, we have to demonstrate that our insight (as shown through reflection) and performance (as shown through behaviour) are improving over time. Because these are fundamental to professionalism and to maintaining fitness to practise, a significant and persistent deficiency in either insight or performance is an early warning that we may be, or may become, a cause for concern. The need to have early warning is critically important to training programmes so that remedial action can be taken.

This competency is concerned with the ability to satisfactorily monitor performance and take action when necessary. The following equation helps us to understand the factors underlying improvement in performance:

d performance =d (insight x motivation x application x opportunity)

d (delta) represents change, reflecting the fact that if the absolute level of performance does not improve with time, in real terms it deteriorates because (to take clinical care as an example) treatment options will improve with medical advances. 'Standing still' therefore translates in the real world as 'going backwards'.

d could be positive or negative. The effects are multiplicatory, not additive, because a zero value in any one of these measures means no (not just less) improvement. We can see that the elements of the equation are not context specific, which means that they can be identified by any observer at any stage of training.

As attributes, we shouldn't think of performance and insight as being separate from each other as the following table explains:

Performance	Insight	Comment
Good	Good	**Ideal**
Good	Poor	**Unconsciously competent**: because the doctor fails to understand why s/he is (currently) competent, the doctor may not adapt to changing situations. The doctor may also engage in risky practices through lack of insight about the connection between action and effects.
Poor	Good	**Consciously incompetent**: the doctor might be difficult to remediate because s/he has low motivation to improve. The causes of low motivation, such as stress need to be looked for and addressed.
Poor	Poor	**Unconsciously incompetent**: this doctor may be the most difficult to remediate because despite regular exposure to deficiencies in performance, s/he may lack the ability to change.

As we can see, we need to both show insight *and* use that insight to improve performance, where this is needed.

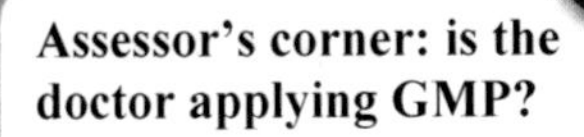

Assessor's corner: is the doctor applying GMP?

Evidence will come from personal observation and from feedback. Does s/he have a mechanism to gauge insight and link this to changes in performance?

How good are the monitoring processes? For example, does s/he recognise the value of data on performance as material that can be used to drive learning?

What range of data does s/he use? This range should include feedback, audit, and the follow-up of cases.

What is the doctor's interpretation of this data; does it show insight and is this level of insight improving over time?

Is personal health discussed? What are the doctor's attitudes to health and work-life balance? What about ethical views?

Are ethical dilemmas recognised and given appropriate thought?

If evidence does not seem to arise naturally, it can be generated through discussion, for example through targeted questioning in CbD.

Our insight can be progressively gauged through frequent opportunistic contacts, particularly through case discussion with colleagues. However, we can and should contribute other meaningful work that demonstrates professional growth beyond evaluations and self-assessment. Examples include:

- Critical incidents of patient events
- Reflective journal or diary
- Clinical care audits
- Articles reviewed using critical appraisal skills

These allow a more substantial opportunity for our insight and critical thinking to be witnessed and they provide evidence of performance in areas that are not easily assessed through the structured tools.

Assessor's corner: how can educators gauge insight?

Insight is an important marker of fitness to practise. When insufficient, it may be an early warning that remedial action is needed

To gauge insight, for example following structured assessments, trainees could explain which competencies in the competence framework they think they are meeting or failing to meet, giving their justification. This could be compared with the views of the educator, looking for significant gaps between the two.

Narrowing of gaps in insight and the gaps in performance related to these, could be looked for over time using evidence from the trainee's completed learning cycles.

Probity: Being honest and trustworthy

Probity means being honest and trustworthy and acting with integrity ,and is at the heart of medical professionalism.

Integrity is a word that is widely used, but what does it mean? Integrity is not a synonym of fairness, but suggests being 'whole' through adhering to an ethical and moral code and of being someone who would not threaten that wholeness by behaving in adverse ways.

The GMC highlight circumstances in which certain action has to be taken if probity is not to be compromised. They say that:

- The GMC should be informed if, anywhere in the world, we have accepted a caution, been charged with or found guilty of a criminal offence
- We must be honest and trustworthy when writing reports, and when completing or signing forms, reports and other documents.
- We must always be honest about our experience, qualifications and position, particularly when applying for posts.
- We must do our best to make sure that any documents we write or sign are not false or misleading. We must make clear the limits of our knowledge or competence.
- We must co-operate fully with any formal inquiry into the treatment of a patient and with any complaints procedure that applies to our work.
- We must disclose to anyone entitled to ask for it, any information relevant to an investigation into our own or a colleague's conduct, performance or health.

Financial and commercial dealings are also part of probity and are mentioned in the chapter on 'maintaining an ethical approach'.

Encourages scrutiny and justifies professional behaviour to colleagues.

If we are performing at the 'excellent' end of this scale, we can demonstrate that maintaining performance is a communal activity. In reality, no doctor can maintain performance in isolation of those around him or her. This is because good insight depends upon high-quality feedback, which is in turn related to high-quality data and to good feedback skills.

To demonstrate this competency, we need to talk about our performance, for example our case management, with colleagues and be proactive in doing so rather than just responding defensively when things go wrong. In practice, 'Justifying professional behaviour' occurs not so much when problems arise as when we share management approaches with colleagues and discuss interesting cases in order to improve our *communal* understanding and insight.

This is particularly important in primary care, where so much of our clinical ability depends upon an understanding of probabilities and an appreciation of what the earliest signs of deviations from an expected path of recovery might look like. Learning from colleagues is therefore invaluable as this allows us to learn from the experience of others, rather than just being reliant upon ourselves.

'Encouraging scrutiny' is qualitatively different. Scrutiny (voluntary or not!) happens routinely during training, because continuous assessment is mandatory. However, *voluntary* scrutiny of performance in independent life is much less frequent and the reasons are understandable. No doctor likes to be seen to perform at a below-average level, let alone poorly. This may be a strong deterrent from being open with others about our 'failures'. The additional complication in practice life is concern about our reputation, in particular the fear of loss of respect from colleagues with whom we have a long-term relationship.

The counterargument to this is that external scrutiny can greatly help us to establish where our weaknesses (and indeed our strengths!) lie. For example, observing consultations through COT can quickly provide objective evidence that can help us to target our learning in a way that self-reflection may not achieve. Far from losing respect, those who encourage such scrutiny are often respected even more by their colleagues for being brave enough to do so and for setting a praiseworthy example of professionalism.

The more that such scrutiny becomes routine, the more that we will see that 'perfect' performance is unattainable and that every doctor has something to learn. In turn, this may help us to have more realistic expectations of each other and encourage us to help each other to maintain performance.

For this competence to be achieved, feedback skills are all-important. It is all well and good exposing oneself to the scrutiny of peers, but if feedback is not given sensitively and formatively, the experience could be damaging, rather than nurturing. Rather than assume that such skills exist, it is better for team members to learn the straightforward principles involved.

Assessor's corner: how can we gauge probity?

Probity has traditionally been demonstrated through self-declaration in NHS appraisal. However, those who work with the doctor are in a position to comment on honesty and trustworthiness as a general feature of the doctor's behaviour and may also be in a position to say whether or not they know of any situation in which this has been breached.

Needs Further Development	Competent for licensing	Excellent
Attends to professional demands whilst showing awareness of the importance of addressing personal needs.	Achieves a balance between professional and personal demands that protects professional obligations and preserves health.	Anticipates situations that might damage the work/life balance and seeks to minimise the adverse effects.

2

This second competency progression is concerned with work-life balance. We move from:

Being dependable with work commitments but not yet thinking seriously about work-life balance.

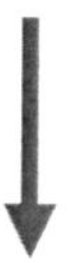

Being dependable with work but at the same time taking active steps to optimise work-life balance.

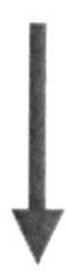

Thinking ahead so that the threats to work-life balance can be identified and reduced.

Looking at each of the word pictures in turn:

Assessor's corner: how do we assess whether the doctor is aware of work-life balance?

The doctor should demonstrate awareness of work-by balance by showing that s/he recognises why the issue is important by talking about personal circumstances and how work and life are in tension with each other and at the same time, are mutually beneficial.

The doctor's attitudes towards work and life should be explored. What is this attitude and is it likely to lead to a healthy or unhealthy balance?

Attends to professional demands whilst showing awareness of the importance of addressing personal needs.

'Doing the job' is the obvious priority and it may seem odd to even be concerned about what we do in our spare time. It may even seem that, provided work commitments are being attended to, what happens outside work is no-ones business but our own.

Why then do we make an issue of work-life balance? Should we live to work or work to live? Here are a few points to help us explore this issue:

Firstly, time and energy are finite and what happens outside work may affect the ability to fulfil practice and other professional commitments. These commitments include the inevitable paperwork generated by patient care (and from which trainees are relatively protected), the time-consuming process of keeping up-to-date through personal study and attending meetings along with the extra time needed to deal with problems and to help develop the practice. Too much time or energy expended elsewhere may limit our motivation or ability to fulfil these responsibilities.

On the other hand, given that doctors are generally highly motivated and tend to work hard without being told do so, there is a risk that time spent on work commitments may seriously limit our ability to engage with the family, develop relationships, develop other interests and take adequate rest. This can lead to physical and emotional problems, as we will discuss later in this chapter.

Work and life need to be in balance because when they are, we feel less stressed and more fulfilled-- as do those who work or live with us. Ask them!

Time spent outside work is time spent in the 'real' world. This helps us to gain vital life experience, which can greatly help our ability to relate to patients and understand their priorities. Because of the length of training we are relatively deficient in personal life experience in our younger years compared to our non-medical contemporaries in society. Therefore, creating time for a 'normal life' is particularly important if we are to gain a balanced view of the world.

When we think about our careers, it is important to think not only about the here and now, but also about how to keep a career sustainable. This has implications for the work-life balance, which if kept under control can help us to prevent burnout. In addition, sustainable careers are usually those that have variety. A good balance allows variety and stimulation from outside sources and helps us to feel fulfilled for a greater proportion of our careers. Examples of ways of achieving work-life balance include part-time and flexible working patterns.

Achieves a balance between professional and personal demands that protects professional obligations and preserves health.

This competency is a step beyond the previous one in that we think about what an adequate work-life balance would be by considering whether the balance is enough to meet work commitments and at the same time maintain physical and mental health. What are the steps involved in this process?

Firstly, we need to think about our current situation. Are work commitments being met? What about life outside the practice? Are important relationships (partner/family) being intended to? These are sensitive areas and although we can answer these questions by ourselves, it is even better to find out what our colleagues and family think. We need to get into the habit of doing this periodically to check on the balance, because such people are much less likely to pretend that everything is okay than we are!

Of course, colleagues and family are likely to always want more from us, but to get the balance right it can be helpful to talk to someone independent such as a friend, colleague, trainer, mentor or appraiser.

Once the current position has been established, the next step is to decide whether any changes in the balance are needed. If this is the case, the obvious step is to the increase the time spent on one by simultaneously reducing the time spent on the other. However if it is possible to be more time-efficient, it may be that the time spent on work can be reduced whilst still meeting the same professional obligations. If efficiency can't be improved, then a reduction in professional obligations may be needed. To do this requires good negotiation skills.

Alternatively, flexible ways of working may help a sustainable work-life balance to be achieved. Here are some examples:

Flexible hours	Simply not having to be at the surgery at 9am can relieve much of the stress of domestic management. Travelling outside the rush hour can take stress out the beginning and end of the day.
Part-time work	Part-time work is particularly beneficial for people with substantial caring commitments, those who are returning to work after looking after young children and those who wish to create time for a portfolio of interests.
Home-based working	Most of us work informally from home but in the future, remote computer access may make this an option for some of our activities, especially consultations that do not require face-to-face meetings. On the other hand, working from home can intrude on family life and may simply lead to taking work home and thereby extending the working day.

Assessor's corner: what is the evidence that the doctor is achieving an appropriate work-life balance?

Assessors could look at a number of areas. 'Protecting professional obligations and preserving health' requires a good deal of insight along with the motivation to repeatedly gauge one's position in relation to these.

To meet this competency, doctors need to engage periodically with colleagues, family and friends and discuss whether the balance is right or needs modification.

Does the doctor discuss these issues? What is his/her assessment of the current balance and on what is this based? How does the doctor maintain work-balance? Is this simply a matter of chance, or does s/he take active steps?

Try posing hypothetical situations (e.g. change of life circumstances/the possibility of a 'special interest' post); how would the doctor address the possible changes to work-life balance?

Anticipates situations that might damage the work/life balance and seeks to minimise the adverse effects.

Assessor's corner: what is the evidence that the doctor anticipates adverse changes to work-life balance?

Doctors who demonstrate this competency are people who think ahead, rather than firefighting when problems arise.

Assessors will only know that this competency is being achieved if the doctor discusses work-life balance issues with colleagues.

Therefore, the doctor must also be someone who communicates well and keeps people in touch with their thoughts about significant changes in their lives.

In addition, these doctors think about themselves in a wider context, looking at the impact of events on others, particularly colleagues and family.

They consult with the others who are affected and are often able to suggest a number of ways forward.

At the 'excellent' end of the scale, we are not only adept at maintaining work-life balance, but can think ahead to situations where this might change.

On the work front, this might occur when there are significant changes in practice that might affect workload such as changes to the service we provide, personnel changes and seasonal variations in workload.

On the home front some 'life changes' will occur that can be anticipated, for example children, family commitments, extramural activities and health issues such as elective surgery.

Career developments can also be anticipated, for example taking on an additional commitment such as becoming a trainer, delivering an extended-hours service or taking on a managerial role.

We can make minimise the adverse effects to our work-life balance in a number of ways such as obtaining advice, getting help (e.g. with childcare) or by altering work commitments. The latter may include simple measures like altering work rotas or more complex ones like renegotiating contracts in order to work flexible hours or take a sabbatical.

Anticipatory action may not simply be the responsibility of the individual. For example, service changes such as offering longer opening hours are likely to affect the work-life balance of doctors, practice nurses and reception staff. Discussing the work-life implications of these changes can help team members decide how the service should be developed and the degree to which they wish to be personally involved.

On a wider scale, doctors may be involved in national negotiations on the terms and conditions of service so that a reasonable work-life balance for *all* doctors can be maintained. An example of this is the way in which GPs lobbied for additional mechanisms of providing out of hours care so that they did not have to be available 24/7.

Needs Further Development	Competent for licensing	Excellent	
Attends to physical or mental illness or habit that might interfere seriously with the competent delivery of patient care.	Proactive in taking steps to maintain personal health.	Promotes an organisational culture in which the health of its members is valued and supported.	3

The third competency progression concerns our personal health and the health of those we are responsible for in the organisation. We move from:

Identifying a personal physical or mental problem and managing this appropriately

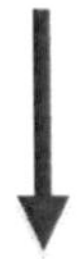

Taking active steps to maintain health, thereby reducing the likelihood of avoidable health problems in the future

Going beyond personal health issues by thinking about the medical and non-medical members of the team and the steps that can be taken to promote health.

Looking at each of the word pictures in turn:

Attends to physical or mental illness or habit that might interfere seriously with the competent delivery of patient care.

Our health matters, because there is little point in achieving competence if our work becomes unsustainable because of health issues.

The first two competencies in this theme are related to each other. To achieve the first, we need to 'attend to illness or habit' in other words, deal with a problem that *already* exists. In the second competency, we act in a preventative capacity by taking steps to maintain our health.

What are the main reasons for early retirement in GPs?

Whilst poor morale and motivation are often given as reasons for leaving medicine, a study of early retirement in the NHS showed that the most common reasons were psychiatric issues such as depression, anxiety and alcoholism.

Not surprisingly, these three are also the most common health issues for doctors.

Time off work

Being doctors does not make us immune to ill health. We are prone to same range of diseases as the general population and would be expected to deal with these in a similar manner to other patients. This is much easier said than done, for a number of reasons:

- GPs have plenty of experience with self-limiting illnesses and may feel that it is reasonable to manage these without seeking independent medical advice. Surveys suggest that two in five of us prescribe antibiotics, painkillers and other medication for ourselves.
- With more significant conditions, we may feel reticent because of practical issues in getting to see a doctor ('there is nobody to cover me if I have to take time off to visit my own GP').
- There may be concerns that confidentiality will not be maintained if ill-health is disclosed, with possible effects on career progress.
- We may be concerned that we will be signed off sick and therefore be unable to work, putting a strain on our colleagues, incurring locum costs etc.
- There is a perceived lack of tolerance towards ill health among doctors. We are 'not allowed to be ill', because it is seen as a form of weakness or liability.
- The occupational health service may be poorly developed and difficult to access.

The literature suggests that we are less likely than other professions to take time off work for ill health. When we are off work, it tends to be for longer periods.

Watch out for burnout!

Burnout describes the syndrome of emotional exhaustion, cynicism, low productivity, and feelings of low achievement. We may think that cynicism is simply a character trait, but some believe that it can be a method of coping with the stress caused by dealing with unmanageable expectations and workload.

If a colleague is frequently cynical, it can be worth exploring stress and workload issues rather than just passing it off.

Dealing with stress

The three most common disorders from which GPs suffer are depression, anxiety and alcoholism, i.e. this doesn't just happen to other people, it happens to us! In doctors, the prevalence is around 20% compared with around 18% in the general working population.

A common cause of these is stress and it is therefore worthwhile for us to know more about stress and how to manage it.

Why is stress increasing? The RCGP offer a useful perspective on this:

'Where GPs would previously accept any professional hardships due to the respect, deference, autonomy and job security offered by the profession, these rewards have now been replaced by greater accountability, a growing blame culture and greater consumer expectation by patients'.

Why are we vulnerable?

GPs become close to their patients, dealing with physical and psychological problems which are often distressing. It can be difficult (i.e. stressful) to maintain an appropriate balance between being empathetic to the patient and sufficiently detached to avoid damaging our health. We may not have the opportunity either at work or at home to debrief or feel adequately supported. In addition, we may exacerbate the problem by being overcritical of ourselves.

What are the main causes of stress for GPs?

Surveys suggest that in descending order of frequency the main stressors are:

- Emergency calls during surgery hours
- Time pressure
- Working after a sleepless night
- Dealing with problem patients
- Worrying about patient complaints
- Interruption of family life (particularly for female doctors)
- Unrealistically high expectations by others of the doctor's role
- Partner on holiday.

Older GPs are more stressed by *contract demands* compared to younger doctors, but younger doctors are more stressed by unreasonable *patient demands*.

If we look at the main causes of stress for GPs we can see that several elements relate to problems with the work-life balance as discussed earlier. Attending to these elements not only helps the balance, but can help to preserve our health.

Wives of GPs are four times more likely to commit suicide than other women, with the main stresses for them being the GPs' detachment from the family, workload concerns and communication problems.

Stress isn't limited to GPs and in fact, we are often the *cause* of stress in other members of the team. Just ask them! A survey of stress in the healthcare team, excluding doctors, suggested that in descending order of frequency the main stressors are:

- Patient demands
- Too much work
- Patient abuse/aggression
- Time pressures concerning appointments
- GP demands
- Poor communication

Team members (unless they have good assertiveness skills!) may feel reticent about discussing the factors that are partly the GP's 'fault'. It is worth asking our team members, whether our behaviour is a significant cause of stress to them and whether there are ways we could change our behaviour. A less stressed and more harmonious team is also likely to reduce the stress on ourselves, so the benefits are two-way.

What are the signs and symptoms of stress to look out for? Again, it is as relevant to look for these in ourselves as in others.

- Lack of concentration, increased errors and adverse significant events
- Poor timekeeping
- Poor productivity
- Difficulty in comprehending new procedures, increased tendency to make mistakes and resisting change.
- Lack of motivation or co-operation along with irritability, aggressiveness, withdrawal behaviour and resentment.

Proactive in taking steps to maintain personal health.

This goes beyond achieving work-life balance. Doctors who achieve this competency demonstrate the ability to think ahead and maintain health, rather than just deal with health issues when they arise. We have illustrated the importance of stress and how it underpins the three most common health issues. Let us now think about how we can be proactive with our health and particularly with managing stress.

How can stress be made manageable?

<u>How can you help yourself?</u>

Here are some practical suggestions. Please think about them.

Registering with a GP

- Register with a GP *before* you need help. It's OK to share information with your colleagues, but not to have informal consultations with them.
- It's important to admit vulnerability. We are human and need support from colleagues and family like anyone else.
- It is much better to behave like any other patient and go through the usual channels. That way, well-meaning but inappropriate shortcuts (like avoiding physical examination) won't be taken and potentially serious problems will not be so easily missed. It's often said that doctors, when they get ill, don't have anything 'straightforward'. Could this partly be because we don't tell anyone early on?
- Remember that the GMC state 'You must ask for and follow your doctor's advice about investigations, treatment and changes to your practice that they consider necessary. You must *not* rely on your own assessment of the risk you pose to patients'

Work & life

- Control the workload. Create appropriate boundaries and don't take on more than you can manage.
- Live healthily, taking the lifestyle advice you give your patients and being careful about alcohol, which is a particular risk for doctors.
- Keep work-life balance under review. It's not just a concept, it's a tool to maintain health, so talk about it periodically. Don't ignore feedback and be prepared to change the balance when necessary.

- Have a life! Make space for yourself; build social networks inside and outside work.
- Make sure that you have activities outside medicine.
- Be organised e.g. make good childcare arrangements, have reliable transport, avoid stressful commutes, arrive with enough time to avoid rushing to catch up throughout the day. Wherever possible, do today's work today so that you are not constantly working to overcome a backlog.
- Give yourself challenges, but not so much as to cause unhealthy stress.
- Make sure you have social support at work. This means investing in your relationship with colleagues and the team.
- Develop stress management skills; there are lots of good resources
- Make sure the work you do continues to have meaning for you. This is vital to maintain motivation over the years.

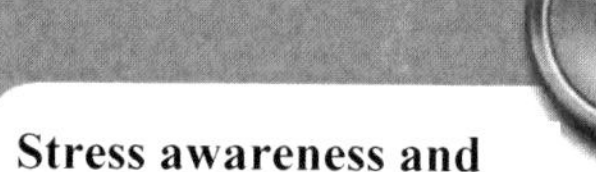

Stress awareness and SWOT analysis

Once we understand more about stress, it can be useful to ask ourselves, 'what are our strengths, weaknesses, opportunities & threats' regarding the stress in our professional and personal lives?

This may help to raise our awareness of areas that we need to attend to and give us ideas on how we might reduce stress before it becomes a problem.

Consulting

Be comfortable and improve the 'feelgood' of the environment that you spend so much time in. For example, look at ergonomics, decoration, personal items and mementos such as a holiday picture on your desktop, photographs and thank you cards in the room.
In surgery, don't be more stressed than you have to be. For example, avoid:

- Starting surgery late
- Overbooking
- Accepting commitments that begin too soon after surgeries are due to finish
- Making insufficient allowances for urgent fit-ins
- Allowing inappropriate telephone or other interruptions in surgery

You don't have to solve these problems on your own. Your manager can help you to achieve much of this.

Keeping healthy and avoiding burnout

- Avoid exhaustion by making sure that you get adequate sleep, periodic breaks, relaxation and regular exercise.
- Deal with problems and with problem people
- Avoid burnout through time management, delegation and being appropriately assertive. LADDER describes a six-stage process for handling problems in an assertive way. These are:

Look at your rights and what you want, and understand your feelings about the situation
Arrange a meeting with the other person to discuss the situation
Define the problem specifically
Describe your feelings so that the other person fully understands how you feel about the situation
Express what you want to say and what you propose clearly and concisely
Reinforce the commitment of the other person by explaining the mutual benefits of adopting the action you are suggesting.

The box describes assertion, not negotiation. GPs are used to negotiation and may find it difficult to be assertive. However an assertive approach can be a fair way of raising and dealing with relationships with people you find difficult and/or powerful. The approach can promote mutual respect because it avoids both inappropriate passivity and inappropriate aggression and allows the facts to be presented relatively dispassionately. This makes it more likely that, through dialogue, a satisfactory solution can be found.

One word of warning: do not apply this approach to problem patients or other vulnerable people to whom you have a duty of care. The situation with them is more complicated and needs to be handled carefully.

Another way of anticipating problems is to complete a questionnaire related to health. An interesting one is MAGPI (Morale Assessment in General Practice Index) authored by McKinstry, Porter, Wrate, Elton &Shaw. An example of a completed questionnaire is shown below:

MAGPI

Please indicate ✓ which statement in each of the following groups best reflects how you feel about yourself and your job ***in the past month:***

A score of **greater than 20** is high and indicates a high possibility of stress. If you have a high score, take time to discuss the issues and think about getting practical help.

Based on the responses shown above, we might reflect on our ratings as shown in the example below:

	Score	**Comments**
1 (a) I feel in control of my work	Control 2	Paperwork is the main problem-this seems to fill the 'gap' between surgeries and isn't getting any better!
(b) Sometimes I find it hard to keep on top of my work ✓...		
(c) I am having great difficulty managing my workload		
2 (a) I get on very well with all my partners ..✓..	Partners 1	My partners are friendly towards me and a recent MSF confirms good relationships.
(b) I am not getting on well with my partners from time to time		
(c) My partners and I do not get on well		
3 (a) I am more up to date with modern practice than the majority of doctors	Up to date 2	I've taken on more duties with teaching undergraduates as a tutor, so I suspect I'm more up to date than the average doctor, but I think that the overall standard for doctors has risen anyway
(b) I am as up to date as most with modern general practice ..✓..		
(c) I have not kept up to date with modern practice		

4 (a) I feel well supported at work ✓ (b) Sometimes I feel a bit let down by the people who work with me ...... (c) I really can't rely on the people I work with to support me	Support at work 1	Generally supportive colleagues and staff, I am fortunate to say
5 (a) I am in good health ✓ (b) I have only minor worries about my health ...... (c) I have been quite worried about my health	Health 1	I play badminton regularly
6 (a) I am well supported at home ...... (b) I could be better supported at home ✓ (c) I have little support at home	Support at home 2	The children are approaching teenage and my wife works part-time as an accountant. She is proud of my new teaching commitments, but I don't think she appreciates the extra demands that this makes on my time. Having said that, I also feel that I haven't the time to support her in ***her*** career
7 (a) I can keep my home life and work in balance satisfactorily ...... (b) It is difficult to keep a balance between work and home life ✓ (c) My work and home life often conflict …...	Work/ Home balance 2	I've had to go to more meetings and have also had to do preparation work in the evenings. As a result, I don't play with the kids as much as I used to. I like to pretend that the kids don't notice, but I'm sure they do.
8 (a) I am a happy person ...... (b) I feel OK but there have been happier times in my life ✓ (c) I am unhappy a lot of the time	Happiness 2	Strange, really. In some ways, things are coming right and my career is developing, but life just seems to get busier. More is not necessarily better.
9 (a) I have family or friends I can turn to ✓ (b) I don't always feel I can turn to friends or family ...... (c) There is no-one I can turn to for help	Help 1	I have a small number of close friends, who I know would listen if I needed it although I try not to bother them.

10 (a) My patients think I do a good job for them ...... (b) I am not sure what my patients think of the job I do for them ✓.... (c) My patients do not value the job I do	Valued by pts 2	I think they probably value me, but I haven't formally asked for some time-maybe I should do another feedback questionnaire.
11 (a) My colleagues generally value me ✓.... (b) I don't know how my colleagues view me ...... (c) I don't think my colleagues value me much	Valued by colleagues 1	They are friendly, but I'm not sure how much they value me as they are not particularly demonstrative.
12 (a) I have no problems with alcohol ✓.... (b) I occasionally wonder if I have become too reliant on alcohol ...... (c) I am worried about my use of alcohol	Alcohol 1	I restrict myself to a glass of wine in the evening and I don't drink & drive. However, I've noticed that my wine glass is a large one.
13 (a) I know that I've chosen the right career ✓.... (b) I quite often wish I had chosen a different career ...... (c) I really regret having chosen my career	Career choice 1	I've never really had any doubts about this. I'm sure that teaching will also increase my job satisfaction.
14 (a) I have no particular worries about my family at the moment...... (b) I have some worries about my family at the moment ✓.... (c) I have serious worries about my family at the moment	Family worries 2	I feel guilty that I'm not pulling my weight at home.
To score the MAGPI, (a) = 1, (b) = 2, and (c) = 3	**21**	
Total score		

Assessor's corner: what is the evidence that the doctor is being proactive about health?

At a basic (but often neglected) level, we might ask whether the doctor has registered with a GP. Does s/he comply with any treatment is required?

Beyond this, what, if anything, does the doctor do to maintain health?

Does the doctor maintain his/her immunisation status? Has the doctor tried to assess risk factors for the work-life balance?

Does the doctor show an awareness of stress? What steps does s/he take to manage stress?

If s/he has had health issues, is there any evidence that these could have been anticipated or prevented?

Learning from MAGPI

Summary

I have a high(ish) overall score, which surprises me. I don't think of myself as being stressed, although I'm certainly busy.
I think that my highest scores reflect the pressure that my work puts on my family priorities. I'm fortunate to be working with enthusiastic colleagues, but that may be part of the problem. We tend to spur each other on and don't particularly talk about achieving a balance.

Issues identified

Getting the work/life balance right. (Could also be an issue for my colleagues generally?)
Being less busy.
Finding out whether my patients value my work.

Learning/ action points

I need to talk to my family and particularly my children. I really don't want to mess things up for our future.
Do less and play more.
Do a patient satisfaction survey.
Possibly raise the 'balance' issue with my colleagues. Perhaps we could share what we have learned from MAGPI?

Changes made

I talked to a clinical lecturer, who was sympathetic and helpful. I was overdoing the preparation for my teaching sessions and probably setting my sights too high. She helped me to set more reasonable goals so that I could have more time with the family.
My colleagues thought that talking about MAGPI was a good idea. We did this in pairs and found that some common themes arose. Even though this did not lead on to any immediate changes, we felt that talking openly in this way was a useful start. I think it has also brought us closer.

Promotes an organisational culture in which the health of its members is valued and supported.

There is an implicit onus on us and other healthcare workers to set a good example by living healthy lifestyles. Doctors who achieve this high level of competence are not only proactive about their own health, but also seek to make health an issue for the team for example by encouraging personal health promotion and by looking at ways in which health could be influenced by the conditions at work.

Why is the health of the team important? Healthy workforces are known to be more productive and to have higher morale, so there are sound *business* as well as compassionate reasons for being proactive. As an employer, there are a number of ways in which the health of the team could be addressed:

- Assess the risk by looking at health and safety issues. These might be physical, such as the risks of strain injuries and infection that could be prevented through ergonomic furniture and appropriate vaccination respectively. Back pain and stress are two very common causes of days lost through illness.
- There may be psychological risks that could be prevented by accessing training on how to manage difficult or violent patients.
- Optimise working conditions (Toilets, space, lighting, temperature) to improve performance by making team members comfortable
- Encourage staff to walk or cycle to work. Provide secure cycle parking, a shower, and encourage physical activity such as charity runs.
- Limit work stress by making reasonable demands and creating an open atmosphere so that problems can be voiced.

- Enable work-life balance rather than assume it. Monitor workloads to keep them sensible, and make sure employees take regular breaks and annual leave so they are getting away from work when they need to.
- Support employees when they become ill. Sick staff often feel under pressure to return to work before they are fully recovered, putting their own health and even the health of colleagues at risk. Stay in contact while they are ill, but do so sensitively. Delegate their work to someone else and reassure them they don't need to return until they are ready.
- Be fair. Make sure that bullying and discrimination are picked up early and dealt with effectively.

We've talked about prevention, but it is worth looking at whether health is *already* a problem. If staff turnover is high or increasing days are being lost to sickness, we should ask ourselves how healthy the workplace really is.

Additionally, 'valuing and supporting the health of the team' also applies to relationships with medical colleagues. Doctors who demonstrate this competence are supportive of their colleagues through a number of mechanisms such as setting a good personal example, encouraging colleagues not to neglect work-life balance/ health and facilitating time off for sickness/medical appointments when this is necessary.

Needs Further Development	Competent for licensing	Excellent	
Notifies when his/her own or a colleague's performance, conduct or health might be putting patients at risk.	Promptly, discreetly and impartially ascertains the facts of the case, takes advice from colleagues and, if appropriate, engages in a referral procedure.	Provides positive support to colleagues who have made mistakes or whose performance gives cause for concern.	**4**

The fourth competency progression concerns the action taken when performance, health or conduct become issues in patient care. We move from:

Being vigilant about performance conduct and health and discussing any concerns before they affect patient care

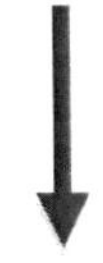

Acting proportionately, collating information and using professional judgement to decide whether a problem or potential problem exists and if so, whether it needs further investigation

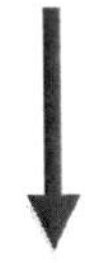

Providing support, but also being constructive in helping colleagues to overcome problems and improve performance.

This progression describes a series of competencies that are not often seen in general practice, or indeed in secondary care. This is partly because these circumstances are (thankfully) rare, but also because the profession is undergoing the culture change that these competencies require. This culture change particularly relates to our willingness to accept joint responsibility for patient safety.

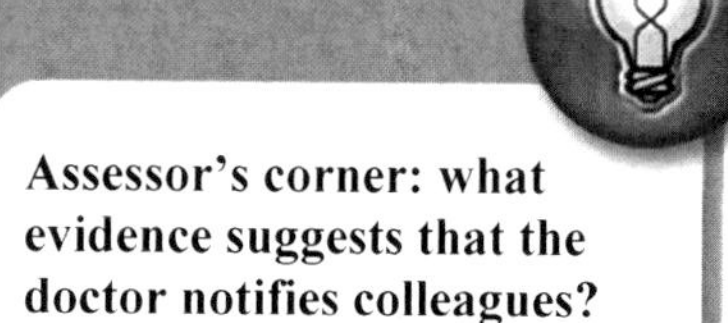

Assessor's corner: what evidence suggests that the doctor notifies colleagues?

Hopefully, the situation may not arise in which patients are put at risk. However, the trainee could be asked what s/he would do in hypothetical situations posed for example in CbD.

Also, how open has s/he been about related matters. e.g. does the doctor talk about *their* health, admit to stress and share how this affects their work?

Another source of evidence is the doctor's learning plan. In effect, this is a notification of an area of performance that needs attention.

How well does the doctor monitor their performance, how proactive is s/he in suggesting learning needs and how much insight into performance do these suggestions show?

Looking at each of the word pictures in turn:

Notifies when his/her own or a colleague's performance, conduct or health might be putting patients at risk.

The previous competency progression concerned personal health and this new theme leads on from this by highlighting the implications for patient safety should personal health become an issue. Beyond health, this competency also describes the action that should be taken if professional performance or conduct put patient safety at risk

This competency does not simply require us to reflect on the issues, but to take personal action. At the 'needs further development' level, we must report the issue to others and at the 'competent' level, we must also take responsibility for looking into the issue and making a judgement on what to do next.

The competencies may sound prescriptive, even intrusive but they reflect the GMC guidance on patient safety, which says the following:

- You must protect patients from risk of harm posed by another colleague's conduct, performance or health.
- If you have reason to believe that patients are, or may be, at risk of death or serious harm for any reason, you should report your concern to the appropriate person or organisation straight away. Do not delay doing so just because you yourself are not in a position to put the matter right.

<u>Obstacles to reporting</u>

During the training period, educators keep trainees' performance under review and therefore performance issues are likely to be noticed. In independent practice this is quite another matter because, legitimately, doctors are not supervised so intrusively. There is therefore a need for us to monitor our own performance and inform colleagues if significant problems arise that they may not be aware of.

Reporting one's own behaviour is difficult, but surmountable. However, reporting the performance of colleagues raises other issues. We may be reluctant to report concerns for a variety of reasons including fear that we might have got it wrong, that reporting will cause problems for colleagues, adversely affect working relationships, have a negative impact on careers or result in a complaint. The GMC remind us that 'if you are hesitating about reporting a concern for these reasons, you should bear in mind that:

- Your duty to put patients' interests first and act to protect them must override personal and professional loyalties.
- The Public Interest Disclosure Act 1998 provides legal protection against victimisation or dismissal for individuals who disclose information in order to raise genuine concerns and expose malpractice in the workplace.
- You will be able to justify raising a concern – even if it turns out to be groundless – if you have done so honestly, promptly, on the basis of reasonable belief and through appropriate channels.

The GMC injunction reminds us that health, performance and conduct are not simply personal issues. However, we are not being asked to behave as 'practice policemen'. In an organisation such as a GP practice, we have a joint responsibility to maintain these three factors at acceptable standards and the way of doing this is by:

- Having a *culture of openness and support* in which health, performance and conduct are talked about routinely rather than just when problems occur.
- *Early, routine notification* of adverse incidents or near misses that allows issues to be addressed, problems rectified and lessons learned without patients coming to any harm. Each such event usually involves several people and systems, not just one 'error'.
- Having enough *information available* so that we can adequately reflect on performance and take action early before significant problems arise
- Having the *personal commitment* to act upon recommendations that are made about our own performance (perhaps through clinical audit) and to check whether the necessary change has occurred.

Raising a concern

The mechanism of raising a concern may be different for doctors in training, but there should be a protocol that provides advice on local procedures. Wherever possible, concerns should be raised with a manager, senior doctor or partner in the first instance. For doctors in training it may be appropriate to raise concerns with a named person in the Deanery.

We should be clear, honest and objective about concerns and when the issue concerns a colleague, we should acknowledge any personal grievance that may arise from the situation and keep the focus on the issue of patient safety.

Professional organisations including medical defence bodies can provide advice on what to do if concerns persist despite notification and it is always sensible to seek such advice before taking further action.

Because this is a complex area with significant implications, it is prudent to keep a record of concerns and any action taken to resolve them.

Promptly, discreetly and impartially ascertains the facts of the case, takes advice from colleagues and, if appropriate, engages in a referral procedure.

This competency moves the game on and is concerned with the performance of colleagues rather than one's own performance. To achieve this level, we must understand and feel comfortable with the idea that good performance is a communal responsibility in which each member of the team must play their part. The competency concerns the practical measures that we take should significant concerns arise.

Because it is highly unlikely that the training doctor will get a real-life opportunity to look into a case where performance, health or conduct is of concern, educators need to think about proxy measures that help to gauge whether the doctor is likely to take the appropriate action should the situation arise. Firstly, let us consider some points relating to the process of investigation.

As suggested earlier, we should seek advice, for example with a senior colleague, before taking any further action.

Assessor's corner: how do we assess whether the doctor is likely to take the appropriate action?

There are three important elements. Firstly, does the doctor understand what action is being expected of him/her?

Secondly, how alert is the doctor to the performance, health and conduct of colleagues? For example, does the doctor (either spontaneously or when asked) comment on the part other doctors have played in the patient's management? Can the doctor give constructive and appropriate feedback on the performance of others?

Thirdly, how appropriate are, or would be, the doctor's actions? For example, where is the doctor's threshold for looking at performance issues in more detail? Do they understand the risks of doing so, as well of not doing so? Do they demonstrate the ability to be discreet, impartial and collaborative when discussing this sensitive area? Is their action proportionate to the problem?

When should we take further action?

The types of behaviour that might trigger action include:

Misconduct, such as misusing information about patients, treating patients without consent, making sexual advances towards patients or otherwise ill-treating them.
Poor performance, such as making serious or repeated mistakes in diagnosing and treating the patient's condition, failing to assess (including examine) the patient properly or not responding to reasonable requests for treatment. Poor performance also includes poor teamwork and poor administration that might compromise patient care.
Criminal or dishonest behaviour in financial matters, in dealing with patients or in research. Behaviour such as driving under the influence of alcohol and viewing illegal Internet sites would also fall under this category.
Physical or mental ill health, including misusing alcohol or drugs, that might put patient safety at risk in situations where the doctor has failed to follow remedial advice.

When would further action not be appropriate?

In some circumstances, the investigating doctor's motivation may be suspect and 'taking things further' would be inappropriate. These circumstances include:

- As a mechanism for addressing personal or practice disputes
- To make a doctor apologise to a patient or professional colleague
- To make a doctor provide a patient with the treatment they want

We need to ensure, through dialogue with colleagues, that any proposed action is justified and does not have some ulterior motive.

What are the characteristics of the doctor that may cause concern?

The comments here should be interpreted with caution as it is important not to be unfairly biased or prejudiced but to take each case on its merits. Feedback from those who deal with poorly performing doctors suggest that there are some personality factors that may predispose to problems. The main ones are:

- Unable to delegate
- Reactive rather than proactive
- Difficulty maintaining relationships
- Unable to team build
- Poor judgement
- Slow learner

Additionally, in recent years doctors who have serious performance issues have been characterised by a combination of common features, principally :

- Professional isolation
- Lack of awareness of their poor performance
- Substantial gaps in their knowledge and skills
- Poor 'people' skills
- Advancing age
- Male sex

This information can help practitioners to be more alert to those colleagues who may require support. If we think of the information as describing the risk factors, it can help us to look for these within ourselves and identify those that might be remediable, for example delegation skills, team working skills and important knowledge gaps.

What action could be taken?

This competency suggests that when faced with a performance issue, we should look 'promptly, discreetly and impartially' into the facts of the case. Our duty is not to conduct an investigation, but to obtain more information on which to base a decision as to whether further investigation is needed. We should then to discuss this information with an appropriate colleague.

In practice, this may mean undertaking some simple checks:

- What are the facts (rather than the rumour)? This may involve looking at the medical records and possibly talking through relevant cases/issues with doctors involved.
- How significant (i.e. serious) is the problem? One way to gauge this is to look at the impact on patient care, particularly patient safety. Has patient harm already occurred, or is it imminent?
- Does this appear to be a one-off or is there evidence that there have been a number of other events that suggest a pattern?
- Is the problem confined to one area of performance, or might there be problems elsewhere? For example, poor interpersonal skills with patients may be mirrored by poor relationships with staff.

Assessor's corner: how can we tell whether the doctor is appropriately supportive?

'Being supportive' can be gauged from feedback received from colleagues and patients. The ability to provide constructive support depends upon the ability to be constructively critical.

A way of assessing this would be to look at the doctor's feedback skills and ability to be both supportive and constructive, rather than just sympathetic.

Provides positive support to colleagues who have made mistakes or whose performance gives cause for concern.

At the excellent end of this competency progression, we not only take personal responsibility for acting upon concerns but show the ability to support colleagues during a difficult period.

The competency is partly about providing emotional support and showing compassion. This may be inferred from teamworking abilities and from feedback from colleagues.

In addition, we should be capable of helping a colleague to develop a plan of action, provide support with implementing it and provide feedback on the changes that the colleague tries to make. The competency talks about doctors who have made mistakes. It therefore means all of us. Because mistakes and significant events are inevitable, we will all need support at some stage of our careers and it's in everyone's interest to make sure that this competency is done well.

Needs Further Development	Competent for licensing	Excellent	
Responds to complaints appropriately.	Where personal performance is an issue, seeks advice and engages in remedial action.	Uses mechanisms to learn from performance issues and to prevent them from occurring in the organisation.	**5**

The final competency progression concerns complaints, what they say or don't say about performance and how the team can learn from them. We move from:

Observing the rules about responding to complaints, using appropriate behaviour when doing so.

Evaluating whether the complaint has implications for personal performance and then taking the necessary steps to change where necessary.

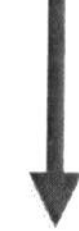

Learning from complaints as a team-based exercise, helping the organisation to become more effective and less error-prone.

Looking at each of the word pictures in turn:

Responds to complaints appropriately.

Sadly, no matter how well we and our practices function, complaints are inevitable in professional life. Patient education and expectations are increasing and the media widely publicise the (comparatively rare) examples of serious issues. These are some of the factors leading to the increase in complaints.

Despite being commonplace, complaints are frequently a source of upset to ourselves as well as those who feel aggrieved. It is best not to take criticism personally as this can adversely affect the response that should be made. For example, we could become defensive or angry, both of which could lead to inappropriate reactions.

Most complaints are dealt with successfully at local level and an appropriate response to a complaint involves a number of steps:

Firstly there are suggested time limits in place for replying to complaints and these should be met. In general practice, the practice manager can make sure of this. Once a complaint is received, there are different approaches for formal (written) and informal complaints with the former requiring a written response and usually needing more investigation and record-keeping.

It is important to deal quickly with the issue and to deal with it positively. Expressing concern and sympathy for what has happened can greatly help. It provides what most patients are looking for, which is to be heard, and is not an admission of guilt or liability.

Once a complaint is received, it can be useful to offer a meeting and give the complainant an opportunity to voice concerns and speak openly and freely without fear of recrimination. It should be made clear that the complaint will be taken seriously, investigated appropriately and that the outcomes will be discussed with the patient. In particular, complainants need to know that *lessons* from legitimate complaints will he learned and changes made so that the chances of recurrence are reduced. This is often a prime motive that patients have when making a complaint. A meeting is also an opportunity to clear the air and to correct any misunderstandings. Showing willing in this way is often enough to stop problems escalating.

Assessor's corner: is the doctor responding to complaints appropriately?

Trainees may not receive any complaints during the training period because of limited patient contact and responsibility, close supervision and perhaps a more forgiving attitude from patients towards students.

However, trainees could talk about how they would respond should complaints arise. What is the doctor's attitude? Is it appropriately constructive?

How would s/he conduct a meeting with the complainant? Role-play could help to disclose this and is good practice for the real thing!

Where personal performance is an issue, seeks advice and engages in remedial action.

Complaints are an important opportunity to look at performance. The *pattern* of complaints may indicate a specific weakness, for example in a clinical area. Communication skills are known to be vital in helping to resolve complaints, but poor communication is itself a frequent source of complaints. When complaints occur more frequently than might be expected, this might point to problems with communication, but may also be indicative of poor health or poor decision-making.

To achieve this competency, we would be expected to use significant events, near misses and complaints as triggers to reflect upon our performance, learning any lessons that may be necessary. The following is an example of a reflection on performance following a written complaint:

Assessor's corner: is the doctor learning from complaints?

If complaints do not arise, there are opportunities through the educational process to gauge whether the doctor is ready to accept negative comments and take remedial action through the learning plan.

When gauging their own performance, does the doctor show adequate insight, avoiding being defensive or (when performance is in fact OK) inappropriately submissive?

The latter is important because doctors must be capable of defending their actions where these actions have been justifiable.

Review of a written complaint	
Date received:	**Outline of the complaint and its background:** A 24 year –old single mum, new to the area and unregistered, rang to sign on and to request an emergency visit for her 3 year old daughter who had a temperature. Mum said she didn't have transport to bring her daughter to surgery and then made out that the daughter was too ill to come anyway. I established that the daughter was not seriously ill and gave telephone advice. Mum took the daughter to casualty, where antibiotics for an ear infection were given, although there were no pathognomonic physical signs. Mum then complained about my 'refusal' to visit. I explained our policy for emergency visits and that lack of transport was not usually an acceptable reason to visit. In the end, the family have decided to register with another practice, which is probably the best outcome for both sides.
Issues arising	Responding to emergency visit requests for new patients who are not familiar with our system. How to handle patients who act unreasonably
Process of resolution/ non-resolution	I was surprised and annoyed by the complaint, as although I had no previous knowledge of the patient I did not refuse to accept her on the list and I did my best to assist her in what she thought was an emergency. I responded by return of post to the complaint, expressing my feelings and my justification for what had been done. I also pointed out that the hospital doctors found no evidence of pathology, supporting my assessment on the phone. I didn't suggest that she register elsewhere, but I was glad that she did as relationships would certainly have been difficult.
Learning points / action points	I may not have been entirely clear about the follow-up arrangements following my telephone advice and this may have led to the patient feeling that I was refusing to visit. I knew that the patient hadn't insisted on a visit and that she seemed to accept the advice, but I had no record of this. In future, I will confirm that the patient accepts my advice before finishing the call and make a note to this effect.
Changes implemented	In future, I'll add a note in my records 'patient happy with the advice given by telephone'

Uses mechanisms to learn from performance issues and to prevent them from occurring in the organisation.

As so often with the descriptors of excellence, the distinguishing feature is that we move beyond our own performance and think about the organisation that we are a part of. As we discussed earlier in this chapter, performance is a communal responsibility. Lessons learned and shared more widely, help the whole team to be more effective and reduce the number of avoidable errors. Cumulatively over time, the impact on patient safety of making lots of little improvements, can be dramatic.

Performance issues, particularly when they lead to significant events such as missed diagnoses, patient harm or complaints, can be important drivers of useful change. The mechanism of conducting significant event review as a team-based exercise that avoids recrimination and maximises learning opportunities, is well described in the books and it should become second nature to us.

Assessor's corner: is the organisation learning from performance issues?

Does the trainee note performance issues and bring them for discussion as SEAs?

Are the lessons that are learned through group discussion then shared with the team? Is there evidence of change in practice behaviour and performance?

Does auditing contribute to this process? How much of a part in this process does the trainee play?

Index

G

H

I

J

L

M

N

O

P

Q

R

S

T

U

V

W